ADOLESCENT PSYCHIATRY

ADOLESCENT PSYCHIATRY

VOLUME 30

THE ANNALS
OF THE
AMERICAN SOCIETY FOR
ADOLESCENT PSYCHIATRY

Lois T. Flaherty

EDITOR

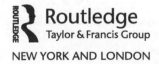
Routledge
Taylor & Francis Group

NEW YORK AND LONDON

ISSN: 0065-2008

Routledge
Taylor & Francis Group
711 Third Avenue
New York, NY 10017

Routledge
Taylor & Francis Group
2 Park Square,
Milton Park, Abingdon,
Oxfordshire OX14 4RN

First issued in paperback 2014

Routledge is an imprint of the Taylor and Francis Group, an informa business

© 2008 by Taylor & Francis Group, LLC

International Standard Book Number-13: 978-0-88163-462-4 (Hardcover)
International Standard Book Number-13: 978-1-138-00592-1 (pbk)

Visit the Taylor & Francis Web site at
http://www.taylorandfrancis.com

and The Analytic Press Web site at
http://www.analyticpress.com

Contents

SECTION III
When clinical skills are not enough: Psychiatric enigmas

Editor's Introduction

The adolescent period of development can be a time of great creativity, as new intellectual capacities come on line, and the adolescent attempts to make sense out of inner and outer experience. The first two chapters in this volume explore adolescent development and creativity. Each takes a different perspective, one examining the adolescent's world view through his creation, while the other looks at an adult's continuing preoccupation with adolescent themes. In the first chapter, Michal Krumer-Nevo looks at the creative production of an adolescent who expressed his anguish over being overwhelmed by sexual and aggressive urges by writing a story that is a recasting of an ancient Greek myth. The choice of a mythological theme is explored and sheds light on the role of myths in articulating basic truths. The story leaves no doubt as to the existence of adolescent turmoil and highlights the fact that it is an internal process not always visible to outsider observers. This teenager used his creativity to master adolescent conflicts and go on to reach adulthood and continue to develop his gifts as a creative writer. The second chapter David Dean Brockman considers evidence of arrested adolescent development in the adult life and art of an extraordinarily innovative artist, Gustav Klimpt. Dr. Brockman, who has studied and written about creativity and adolescence, discusses Freud's and his own views on creativity.

Adolescent psychiatry has never been easy, but it seems to be getting harder. Adolescent psychiatrists observe that the patients we see today are more disturbed than those seen in clinical settings in the past. Studies done in the U. S. have been inconclusive (Roberts, Attkisson, and Rosenblatt, 1998), but these studies have been plagued by methodological problems. A carefully done research study in the United Kingdom confirmed that the prevalence of problems with behavior and emotions among young people there is increasing, and that the increase is not simply the result of differences in threshold for identification or changes in diagnostic criteria (Collishaw, Maughan, Goodman et al., 2004). This study showed a substantial increase in the prevalence of adolescent conduct problems from 1974 to 1999. The rate more than doubled, going from approximately 7% to nearly 15%. The increase affected males and females, and all social classes and all family types. There was also evidence for a recent rise in emotional problems (measured as worry, misery, and fearfulness in new situations), but mixed evidence in relation to rates of hyperactive behavior. It is intriguing that the conditions most linked to parenting and social context showed the most dramatic change, while hyperactivity, presumably more biologically based, did not increase, and those that are probably influenced by both environment and genetics (mood and anxiety) were in the middle.

It seems likely that these findings would be replicated in North America if the same methodology were to be used. Although isolating the causes of the increasing prevalence is a daunting prospect, genetic causes can be ruled out, as 25 years is too short a time for them to have a significant population impact. This leaves environmental factors. Not many people think that these are related to something in the water—most agree that they consist of the social and family contexts in which children grow up. Exactly what these environmental risk factors are remains to be demonstrated in rigorous studies, but no less a researcher than Michael Rutter, drawing on a lifetime of studying epidemiology and risk and protective factors, considers that the many stresses of contemporary life are to blame. These include the widespread availability of recreational drugs, increasing prevalence of divorce, lengthening of the adolescent time period, increasing freedom of adolescents to make their own decisions about sexuality and intimate relationships, increased emphasis on educational attainment, low-quality child care during early childhood, and increasing socioeconomic disparities (Rutter and Smith, 1995). In addition there are the influences of the media, youth culture, and degree of social cohesion in adolescents' milieus. To compound the difficulties, clinicians are faced with ever-increasing hurdles to providing good care— insufficient funding for treatment, closing of facilities, and too few well-trained mental health professionals, especially psychiatrists, who can work effectively with adolescents.

In light of all this, can there be any question but that adolescents need "saving"? Thus it is appropriate that Richard Rosner, in receiving the Shonfeld Award at the 2005 ASAP Annual Meeting, titled his address, reprinted here, "Saving Adolescents." Speaking on the basis of his life's work in forensic psychiatry, and as a psychiatric educator, as well as a more recent interest in addiction medicine, he summarizes his perspective on what is needed to help troubled adolescents. He advocates for better treatment of youth with substance abuse problems and those in the juvenile justice system, and more training in adolescent psychiatry for general psychiatrists.

The remainder of the special section in this volume, Difficult Challenges— Creative Solutions, attempts to address many of the more daunting challenges in adolescent psychiatry through describing creative and novel approaches to difficult clinical and service delivery situations.

Adolescents who commit sex crimes are a particularly challenging group, not well studied. Many are in the public sector as they enter through the criminal justice system. The financially strapped public sector is not an environment particularly conducive to conducting research. In addition, confidentiality issues must be considered. Dwyer and colleagues describe an approach to assessment of juvenile offenders as well as data collection based on their use of standardized data collection at the time of entry into the system to determine demographic profiles and clinical needs.

Three chapters by Thomas Bratter and Lisa Sinshimer focus on an innovative residential treatment program for gifted adolescents who have failed academically and rejected previous attempts at treatment. In doing so, they highlight the failures of much of contemporary mental health treatment, which, failing to consider the context in which disruptive behavior occurs, labels acting-out teenagers with a multitude of psychiatric diagnoses, and medicates them in an attempt to control their behavior. These authors view medication and diagnoses as "excuses" that prevent youngsters from assuming responsibility for their actions. While controversial, their anti-medication stance makes sense for this particular group of teenagers, many of whom probably have personality disorders and conduct disorders, and who have the capacity to succeed if they can be motivated. The authors present impressive results in terms of their graduates' success at college.

Motivational interviewing lies at the opposite end of the spectrum from confrontation. At the heart of it is finding a common ground between the therapist and patient where both agree on what needs to be changed. My chapter on this technique grew out of curiosity about it after hearing a presentation by Richard Rosner on approaching substance abuse in adolescents. While originally developed in the 1980s to treat substance abuse in adults, motivational interviewing has received renewed attention in recent years, and has been adapted for a variety of risk-taking behaviors in adolescents. It can be easily incorporated into psychotherapeutic work.

The increasing prevalence of divorce is a fact of contemporary society and a risk factor for children and adolescents, especially when there are conflicts over custody. Helping adolescents to articulate their own preferences, making recommendations to the court that will maximize likelihood of the teenager's continuing to maintain a bond with both parents, and providing valuable information to the family court judges about what is in the adolescent's best interest, can reduce risk to adolescents who are caught in the middle of messy divorces. Harvey Feinberg brings to bear a wealth of clinical experience in describing how he approaches these difficult situations as a consultant to the court, and gives us many clinical pearls as he describes the role of a forensic consultant in contested custody cases.

Despite our acknowledgement of the importance of sexuality in human life in general, and its particular salience for adolescent development, we actually know relatively little about it. Whether or not an adolescent has had sexual intercourse—a fact that most of us routinely inquire about in our assessments—tells us little about the most important aspect of sexual experience: what it means to the adolescent. Important dimensions of adolescent sexuality include mutuality, emotional maturity, quality of interpersonal relationships, capacity for intimacy, and sense of self. To understand these larger issues, we need to inquire about the meaning of sexual experience and sexual feelings for the adolescent. Ashley Harmon, in a paper that won the 2006 ASAP award for best paper by a psychiatric resident, discusses the importance of taking a sexual history and offers guidelines on how to go about it, suggesting that discussing sexual side effects of medications with adolescent patients, something that is not generally done well, can facilitate self-disclosure of sexual concerns and lead to meaningful work with the adolescent.

The third section in this volume deals with two disorders that present major challenges to our clinical skills, reactive attachment disorder and schizophrenia. These chapters reflect the fact, I believe, that we are setting our standards ever higher in terms of what we try to do. We now routinely treat as outpatients many adolescents who would have been hospitalized or in residential treatment for 1–2 years in the past. We try to help children who have been severely emotionally damaged since infants adapt to adoptive families. We expect that adolescents with biologically based brain disorders such as schizophrenia and bipolar disorder, or those with substance abuse, will have a good enough response to treatment to be able to return to school and live in the community. We have an impressive armamentarium to offer these patients. And they often make astonishing progress. But this is not always the case.

The diagnosis of reactive attachment disorder has been controversial in adolescents. Originally meant to apply only to young children, with the increased prevalence of adoptions of older children who were raised in orphanages under conditions of extreme deprivation, it became clear that mainly of the problems manifested by older children could be traced to attachment problems. John Kemph and Kytja Voeller review the literature on this challenging disorder and offer an intriguing hypothesis on possible genetic vulnerability to explain why some children seem permanently damaged by early lack of parenting and others seem resilient enough to bond with adoptive parents or other caretakers. They then present cases that demonstrate disparate outcomes and speculate on what might account for the differences.

While new antipsychotics hold promise, they don't always work. Stahl and colleagues describe two cases of treatment-resistant schizophrenia in adolescents and remind us that this illness can be particularly pernicious in adolescents, despite advances in psychopharmacological treatment. Max Sugar, in his discussion of their chapter, wonders if anything else could have been done and whether all the pertinent psychosocial factors were addressed. The authors respond by reminding us that our patients don't always improve, even with our best efforts, and in state-of-the-art facilities. These chapters underscore the fact that much remains to be done, with respect to both the art and the science of adolescent psychiatry.

References

Collishaw, S., Maughan, B., Goodman, R., & Pickles, A. (2004), Time trends in adolescent mental health. *J. Child Psychol. Psychiatry*, 45:1350-1362.

Roberts, R. E., Attkisson, C. C., & Rosenblatt, A. (1998), Prevalence of psychopathology among children and adolescents. *Amer. J. Psychiat.*, 155:715-725.

Rutter, M. & Smith, D. J. (1995), *Psychosocial Disorders in Young People: Time Trends and Their Causes*. Chichester, UK: John Wiley & Sons.

About the Authors

Jonathan Steven Alter is a houseparent at the John Dewey Academy in Great Barrington, Massachusetts and a college student at Yale University, New Haven, Connecticut.

Carl C. Bell, M.D. is President and Chief Executive Officer of the Community Mental Health Council, Inc., Chicago, Illinois, and Professor of Psychiatry and Public Health, at the University of Illinois at Chicago.

Thomas Edward Bratter is President and Founder of The John Dewey Academy in Great Barrington, Massachusetts.

David Dean Brockman is Clinical Professor of Psychiatry at the University of Illinois Medical School in Chicago and Training and Supervising Analyst at The Institute For Psychoanalysis of Chicago.

R. Gregg Dwyer, M.D., Ed.D. is Assistant Professor in the Department of Neuropsychiatry and Behavioral Science at the University of South Carolina School of Medicine and Director of the Sexual Behaviors Evaluation, Research and Treatment Clinic and Laboratory at the University Specialty Clinics, Columbia, South Carolina.

Harvey Feinberg, M.D. is Assistant Clinical Professor of Psychiatry at Mount Sinai Medical School and a Forensic Consultant in New York City.

Lois T. Flaherty, M.D. is Adjunct Associate Professor at the University of Maryland School of Medicine and Editor of Adolescent Psychiatry.

Richard L. Frierson, M.D. is Associate Professor of Clinical Psychiatry and Director of the Forensic Psychiatry Fellowship in the Department of Neuropsychiatry and Behavioral Science at the University of South Carolina School of Medicine in Columbia, South Carolina.

Ashley Harmon, M.D. is a Clinical Instructor at Harvard Medical School and a member of the teaching faculty at Cambridge Hospital in the Division of Child and Adolescent Psychiatry in Cambridge, Massachusetts.

Margaret E. Hertzig, M.D. is Professor of Psychiatry and Interim Vice-Chair of Child and Adolescent Psychiatry at Weill Medical College of Cornell University, New York.

Danielle Sara Kaufman is a Clinical Psychology Ph.D. candidate at Yeshiva University in New York City.

John P. Kemph, M.D. is a child and adolescent psychiatrist in a solo office practice in Scottsdale Arizona, and a psychiatric consultant to mental health treatment centers.

Michal Krumer-Nevo, Ph.D. is a Lecturer in the Spitzer Department of Social Work, and Academic Coordinator at The Israeli Center for Qualitative Methodologies, at Ben-Gurion University of the Negev, Beer-Sheva, Israel.

Richard Rosner, M.D. is Clinical Professor of Psychiatry at the New York University School of Medicine, Director of the Forensic Psychiatry Residency at the New York University Medical Center and Medical Director of the Forensic Psychiatry Clinic, Bellevue Hospital Center.

Theodore Shapiro, M.D. is Professor Emeritus in Psychiatry at Weill Medical College of Cornell University, New York.

Lisa Sinsheimer, M.D. is a psychiatric consultant and Admissions Coordinator at The John Dewey Academy in Great Barrington, Massachusetts.

Atara S. Stahl, M.D. is a Fellow in Child and Adolescent Psychiatry at Payne Whitney/New York Hospital-Cornell Medical Center, New York.

Max Sugar, M.D. is Emeritus Professor of Clinical Psychiatry at Louisiana State University Medical Center in the Department of Psychiatry, and Professor of Clinical Psychiatry at Tulane University Medical Center in the Department of Psychiatry, New Orleans, Louisiana. He is also a Past-President of ASAP and was Editor-in-Chief of Adolescent Psychiatry from 1982-85.

Wendy Turchin, M.D. is a Child and Adolescent Psychiatrist and Assistant Professor of Psychiatry at Weill Medical College of Cornell University, New York.

Kytja K. S. Voeller, M.D. is a Pediatric Neurologist and Program Director of the Western Institute for Neurodevelopmental Studies and Interventions in Boulder, Colorado.

Johnny L. Williamson, M.D. is Director of the Disruptive Behavior Disorders Clinic at the Community Mental Health Council Inc. in Chicago, Illinois and the Owner of Williamson Health Associates Inc., a Private Practice in Chicago.

Section I

Adolescent development and creativity

1 Mythology, sexuality, aggressiveness
Adolescence and creativity

Michal Krumer-Nevo

Abstract

This chapter presents a short story written by a 15-year old boy as a startling response to a regular class assignment. Its originality and the expressive emotional and experiential power of the writing make it an exceptional text, worthy of close analysis. The story, based on *The Odyssey*, follows the life of Cyclops Polyphemus*—from his childhood, through the recognition of the mature body and especially the "eye," the cannibalistic scene at the cave, and the blindness.

By choosing a story so distant from human reality and using the mythological giant-monster figure protagonist as a model for identification, the adolescent author succeeds in evoking the world of adolescent feelings and the power of its sexual fantasies, anxieties, desires, and frustrations. The analysis of the story is based on the following concepts: psychological birth, masturbation fantasy, primal scene, and castration fear. Through the analysis, the process of adolescence as the psychological birth of the sexual body is unfolded.

Introduction

Special difficulties face research that is focused upon adolescence. Anna Freud (1958) ascribed these difficulties to the extremely high level of emotional sensitivity to the world and the self characteristic of the stages of puberty. The adolescent experiences a very rich repertoire of intense emotions too powerful, and often too painful, to be easily dealt with in psychotherapy during adolescence or to be reconstructed in adult analysis. However, these emotions and experiences are sometimes expressed by gifted adolescents through artwork (Rakoff, 1993). These artworks serve as a mode of knowing, of self-expression and interpersonal communication, and are a rich source for the understanding of adolescent experiences. My intention in this article is to use a literary work—a short story written by a 15-year old boy—as an aid to understanding some aspects of the elusive occurrence in our lives that we call adolescence.

---

* The Cyclops were a race of huge one-eyed monsters who resided on an island with the same name. Commonly, the name "Cyclops" refers to a particular son of Poseidon and Thoosa, named Polyphemus, who was a Cyclops. Cyclops Polyphemus was blinded by Odysseus to enable Odysseus's escape from the cave in which the Cyclops had trapped him and his men.

The story was written in response to a class assignment to write a story on any subject. After its return to the author, the story lay forgotten in a drawer for many years. More than 10 years later I became acquainted with the author, now a grown man, and in the course of the friendship that developed between us he showed me the story. He also approved of my publishing it together with the interpretation.

The story, which takes the form of a dream-narrative, is based on the Cyclops episode in *The Odyssey*. By choosing a story so distant from human reality and using the mythological giant-monster figure protagonist as a model for identification, the adolescent author succeeds in evoking, while distancing, the world of adolescent feelings and the power of its sexual fantasies, anxieties, desires, and frustrations. It is not my intention in this article to come to any predictive or clinical conclusions concerning the life experiences of the young writer, whose literary talent continued to develop through his adult life. My analysis refers to the narrative simply as a paradigmatic expression of certain adolescent state of mind.

The story, entitled "Cyclops Polyphemus", was written originally in Hebrew, and was translated for the purpose of this article, making every effort to keep the style and level of language usage.

The first part of the article contains the story. It is followed by a brief review of the literature and my interpretation, which makes use of the concepts of psychological birth, masturbation fantasy, and castration fear.

Cyclops Polyphemus—The Story

These are the generations of Cyclops Polyphemus. On the first day Cyclops Polyphemus was lying on the ground on the island of the sun, his feet buried in the sands of the sea, his head resting on the great plains.

On the second day, Cyclops Polyphemus was seated on the sand, his hands joyously sprinkling water about. Cyclops Polyphemus was rather plump.

On the third day Cyclops Polyphemus sat up and scratched his back against the mountains and read a nice story about a one-eyed monster who ate human beings. On the first day Cyclops Polyphemus was stretched out, breathing and steamy on the hot earth. The touch of the sun's rays was pleasant and the touch of the waves of the sea was pleasant. Cyclops lay and lay upon his back. His hand stretched out and fingered his forehead until something his fingers touched made them draw back. Cyclops smiled.

Again his hand stretched out and advanced slowly and cautiously over what he had touched—his eye. A tremor seized his body. The eye's cornea was smooth and very polished and shiny. The face of Cyclops Polyphemus was coarse and hot but his eye was smooth and cool. It was a large eye, the size of the palm of Cyclops Polyphemus's hand. It was an eye of a strange green-blue glittering color. It was round and big and fixed in the forehead of proud Cyclops Polyphemus. It was a thick eye, prominent upon the forehead of Cyclops Polyphemus like a deep glass ball whose color shifted back and forth between dark green and light blue. A finger of Cyclops wandered over the jellied lump that was cold and rubbery. His member* stretched and enlarged and a stream of liquid pushed and poured out, its drops disappearing in the shining sky through which they fell.

Cyclops Polyphemus loved the sea. In his spirit he floated with dancing steps over the sea's surface, his neck erect and proud, a thin, hidden smile upon his face.

On the fourth day Cyclops ran peacefully in the fields hopping from side to side, and climbed the tree and hid among the branches and the leaves of the tree. Only his scared, wondering face could just be discerned among the branches and the leaves of the tree. Soon Cyclops gobbled up all the leaves, leaving the branches bare. Then his round, wondering face was revealed and the soft limbs of his body. Cyclops stood up at his full height and thrust his elongated head towards the sun. His figure was formed wonderfully well with its stretched neck and straight chin jutting out diagonally upwards. He blew soap bubbles, slowly, from a hollow tube. Bubbles, completely round, smooth and light, floating. Bubbles fracturing the light into colors. The bubbles moved with the eddies of air: there were some balls, light and transparent, which burst. But there were some balls, light and transparent, which rose up to the sun. Cyclops stared a long time at the sun. He felt its heat, and wanted to grab it, and to put it on his tongue.

Cyclops was sturdy. His hair was shorn right down to the roots. He plummeted to the earth like a mast, stricken and sinking. His arms were spread out to the side but the front of his body was hard and the earth trembled. Cyclops sank his colored nails into the earth. He pushed and shoved. He dug, and barked angry barks and thrust his head into the earth. The earth was warm. He lay thus many years.

Cyclops Polyphemus fell upon the patches of thick green grass and ate them. He opened his mouth and his white teeth chewed the earth. He munched lumps of soil and crushed the stones that wrestled with his white teeth. Behind the thigh of the mountain he saw a lit up green expanse and ran, hopping, trampling and kicking over the deep holes, assailing the grasses and the thorns, his mouth biting with hasty, sudden movements. His roars swallowed up the desert's clamor. He loved to eat the lumps of earth and the grains of sand, and he loved the sour-bitter taste of the herbs and the grasses, and the thorny plants and the young trees and the bushes. On the morning of the fourth day Cyclops got up and stretched himself with a sigh beneath the heavens. He hummed a song he had composed himself:

There was a man from the land of Oz
Toodly pim pam pom

---

* The Hebrew word *ayvar*, used by the author in the original text, is a literary euphemism for "penis".

There was a man from the land of Oz
Toodly pim pam pom
There was a man from the land of Oz
Toodly ly ly ly.
And he was called Utzly Gutzly!*

Cyclops loved the word "Gutz" very much. From his huge mouth, from the cave of his red jaw, escaped all kinds of whistles, and grunts and snorts and roars. He sang the song again and emitted a hoarse joyful shout: There was a man from the land of Oz toodly pim pam pom, until his voice broke and became a thin screech, and then he got up and looked around threateningly and in dread.

He came to the cave and found there the accursed invaders: human beings, small and cute. They were alarmed at the sight of him. Cyclops Polyphemus was hungry. The song had increased his hunger. With his hands he grabbed two of the humans. He stared at them a long time. He enjoyed seeing the eyes and the noses and the mouths and the ears and all the details of their tiny bodies. He enjoyed seeing their shapely delicate bodies. He yelled with delight when he discovered their miniature genitals. Suddenly his hand whipped out and tore off the two sexual organs. His huge laughter cascaded at the sight of their horrified wide open eyes and gaping mouths. He chewed up the bits of soft meat. His reddened teeth were visible. An obscure excitement seized Cyclops Polyphemus. He had two trembling warm bodies upon his tongue. He split them and crushed them with his teeth and felt the drops of the new, enchanting tastes. He drank their blood and their blood quenched his ancient thirst. He gnawed and sucked the brittle, succulent bones, swallowed the moist, warm, sweetish, melting meat. Only the heads he didn't like, so he spat out the hairy skulls. Now he hated earth, its stones and grasses and its grains of sand and its thorny plants. Cyclops Polyphemus lay down full of happiness and slept a misty sleep, his hand stroking and caressing the small, cute humans. His eye was open, and as fine and clear as ever. In his dream he saw the small humans grasping, all of them together, the trunk of a tree, swinging it upwards, approaching at a run and plunging it into his repulsive eye, his beautiful eye. He was shocked, fumbling, toppling, seizures tore through his big body, his nails scraped at the black stone walls. The people raced between his trembling legs. Their laughter was light and clear. He staggered outside into the obscure brightness, dragging his feet. Blind.

Cyclops Polyphemus ran slowly, tottering from side to side, bending towards the flowers, until he reached the tree, climbed up it and sat among its foliage. He wrinkled his brow, shaded his eye with his hand, and contemplated his surroundings. He heard the voices of the people from within the mountain. He tore out a lump of rock. Above his head his two hands stretched tight around the piece of rock. He hurled it into the Atlantic Ocean, for while he was performing

---

* Utzly Gutzly is the Hebrew translation of Rumpelstiltskin, from the Grimm Brothers' tales.

all his high deeds the people had surrounded his island in their ships, threaded their way between the Cyclades, sailed past Crete, raced towards the Ionian Isles, crossed through the Straits of Messina, hurtled past the Liparian Islands, wandered in the Tyrene Sea, slipped through the Bonifacio Straits, and dodged between the Belarian Isles, bobbing and swaying in the fierce storms. But once they had passed Alborn they hurried to make their way into the Great Sea as they forced a passage through the dangerous waters of the Straits of Gibraltar. And Cyclops Polyphemus heaved the mountain of stone into the Alantic Ocean, his wild scream accompanying the huge cliff cutting through the air in a whistling arc, threatening in the skies of the world, till he heard the sound of cracking wood and the thunder of wreckage and the roar of huge waves. That was the swan song of Cyclops Polyphemus. He stood and dreamt. He dreamt that he rolled, fainting, into the cave. People whispered in the depths of the cave. The light of a small fire alternately illuminated and shadowed their faces. Strong, determined faces. People are racing in the dream. In the dream the trunk of a tree is red and hissing. People make dance steps, full of grace. In the air. Their hands wave in the air. They hold their heads high. A faint smile on their faces, mysterious and arrogant. Now they kneel and pray. Suddenly they surround the reclining Cyclops Polyphemus in a circle. Their faces and bodies are colored in hideous colors. They jerk from leg to leg with loathsome heaviness. Their faces express a frozen mirth. They roll about on the ground like thrown away elastic dolls, their hands on their stomachs. Laughter prostrates them. One points to him and the throttled laughter bursts out and swells. Cyclops Polyphemus gets up and begins confidently to walk. His feet feel their way and lead him, but suddenly he loses his balance and he begins slowly to roll over. The black air is dense and soft. He turns away his head.

In the dim light between the trees he sees the figure of a ridiculous giant. The figure stoops forward in great concentration. Its face is pale, its hands harden over the ground. Its legs are bent in the posture of a leap, pressed against the blocks. He awaits a sign. The flexible, supple and tough body seems to freeze, to solidify in its obstinate posture of withheld ominous power. He awaits a sign. Every nerve in his body is ready, his muscles tense and aching. He waits for some sign. Strange creaks are heard from his broken back. His muscles are about to tear. He stops and awaits a sign. At last Cyclops sees the face that is turned to the ground slowly raised, a tormented face, saturated in reproof. Cyclops studies the face with great interest, unable to tear his gaze away from the gaping black hole in the middle of the forehead.

Cyclops Polyphemus turned over on his stomach. He buried his mangled forehead in the earth and lay quiet until he stretched out his arms and crammed the nails of his hands and his toenails into the ground. His hands and knees pressed into the ground, penetrating ever deeper and deeper. They dug into the warm earth. Cyclops trembled, mad Cyclops upturned the patch of earth on which he lay and he glided and slithered into the vale of earth. The heavy, dense, moist earth covered him. The intense heat was very pleasant to him.

Adolescence as the psychological birth of the sexual body

This story is an unusual manifestation of creativity during adolescence. The main characters described in the story, the plot, and especially its emotional intensity, reveal a turbulent inner world, highly personalized. Understanding the story, therefore, requires a readiness to read it as a set of symbols and metaphors. The most prominent characteristic of Cyclops Polyphemus is his loneliness. Before the invasion of the small human beings, his world is empty. His mother and father, siblings, and friends are absent, signifying the experience of facing an extreme crisis in isolation. His modes of relating to others (beside the episode in the cave) cannot be deduced from the story. At the same time, I would argue, the story can be understood as a story of adolescence, expressing vividly some of the conflicts and experiences of that phase.

The central psychosocial task of adolescence is the process of identity formation, which occurs through the acceptance of bodily changes as well as of new libidinal feelings and by the choice of an ideology or philosophy of life, a vocational preference, religious affiliation, forms of friendship, loyalty, and sexual orientation and behavior (Erikson, 1965). Using Freedman's (1968) term, adolescence is "obsessed" by puberty. Its major tasks are (a) the establishment of the final sexual organization and of body representation, which includes the physically mature genitals and the changing body; and (b) libidinal detachment from parental figures in order to find new sexual objects outside the family (S. Freud, 1953; Blos, 1967; Laufer and Laufer, 1984). This process, "by its nature an interruption of peaceful growth" (A. Freud, 1958, p. 275) is, in other words, a crisis. It entails manifest temporary id and ego regressions, changes in the uses made of identifications, and alterations in the types of object relations (Laufer, 1966). Yet, in an optimally successful process the adolescent eventually attains a subjective sense of comfort with the body, the self, and others.

Cyclops Polyphemus is a narrative of crisis and of beginning. It is a narrative of an active identity search (Erikson, 1968) or a narrative of what I shall call, paraphrasing Mahler (1975), "the psychological birth of the sexual body." While more than one theorist of adolescence has implicitly drawn upon analogies to birth, Mahler speaks explicitly of a birth process: "The biological birth of the human infant," she says, "and the psychological birth of the individual are not coincident in time. The former is a dramatic, observable and well-circumscribed event; the latter is a slowly unfolding intra-psychic process" (p. 3).

As in birth itself, adolescence, as exhibited in Cyclops Polyphemus, is the dramatic climax of the stubborn, painful process of severance from the womb, or its symbolic continuation, threatening even as it protects. By using the biblical formula, "And these are the generations of Cyclops Polyphemus," we are already at the beginning of the story in the presence of an act of genesis; the psychological birth of the mythological creature resembles the mythological creation of the world and of mankind. Cyclops Polyphemus is indeed very like a human being. In the first days he is a happy child. He is plump, innocent, and lovable. He eats grass and plays games. Nature exists in order to serve him and provide him with support, the sun warms him and protects him like a holding mother: "On the first day Cyclops Polyphemus was lying on the ground on the island of the sun, his feet buried in the sands of the sea, his head resting on the great plains. On the second day Cyclops Polyphemus was seated on the sand, his hands joyously sprinkling water about." The harmony with nature and the perception of the world as a field full of games and surprises reminds us of Mahler's (1975) symbiosis stage. In its optimal state it is characteristic of a happy and secure childhood. So, too, is the omnipotence which is implied in the description. The universe and all its contents are at his disposal while Cyclops Polyphemus is protected by his enclosure within a huge, calm, and supportive world.

The first hint of changes that are about to occur comes through the cognitive or intellectual act of reading. As part of his playing, Cyclops reads of a one-eyed monster that eats human beings. This is the first time in the story that creatures other than Cyclops himself or any interaction between any other creatures is mentioned. The reading about the one-eyed monster leads him to touch, and so discover as if for the first time, the protuberance on his forehead: "Cyclops lay upon his back. His hand stretched out and fingered his forehead until something his fingers touched made them draw back. Cyclops smiled." The smile is the expression of an insight, a first recognition of his identity as a Cyclops, one of those monsters whose adult task is to devour human beings.

The single eye in the story thus serves two purposes. Metaphorically it is the symbol of the penis—both the eye and the penis are single organs, not one of a pair; both are positioned in the middle of the body (or the face), in the center, and are providers of pleasure. But an eye has a literal meaning: it is the organ of looking, seeing, the organ of knowledge and consciousness. The meanings converge. The penis thus becomes the critical organ of a new consciousness of oneself and of the world. It is the eye/penis which is the tool of connection both to the self and to the outer world and its tasks. By fulfilling the role of the penis, the Cyclops/child will supposedly gain his new identity as an adult Cyclops, or as a man.

It is interesting to note that in this story the first stage in the growth of awareness of the penis arises from an external cognitive stimulus, and the bodily experience follows. The reading of the story awakes in Cyclops the latent, incipient consciousness which leads him to caress his forehead. That caress of the eye, the first masturbation, is almost fortuitous, although the minute it happens it seems right, as if this is something the Cyclops ought to do, part of his destiny. The discovery of the pleasure and the mission of the "eye," as a consequence of reading the book about the monster, can be compared to a child's knowledge of mature sexual life. The knowledge remains detached from any sense of a sexual function the child will one day take upon him/herself to perform. It is not before adolescence—when a certain degree of physical, emotional, and cognitive maturity is arrived at—that the child, now a youth, understands the meaning of what is being read or shown, and its implications for him/herself.

Cyclops smiles in response to his discovery of the eye. He is happy and proud of the discovery he has made and checks it once again out of pleasure and curiosity. "Again his hand stretched out and advanced slowly and cautiously over what he had touched—his eye. A tremor seized his body." "A finger of Cyclops wandered over the jellied lump that was cold and rubbery. His member stretched and enlarged and a stream of sticky liquid poured out, its drops disappearing in the shining sky through which they fell." This first masturbation signifies the onset of Cyclops's active journey into adolescence. After the discovery of the genitals and the pleasure they provide, childhood is over, even though Cyclops is not ready for or desirous of its termination. The first masturbation causes the arousal of anxiety and the weakening of defenses (Laufer and Laufer, 1984). The story that unfolds hereafter is the story of the anxious Cyclops, who tries vigorously and helplessly to cope with the new body and its feelings.

By acknowledging the mature body and bodily feelings, primary resolution of the oedipal love, and former defenses used in this regard, are endangered (Laufer and Laufer, 1984). In the story the first masturbation causes the onset of dramatic turmoil which includes two phases. The first phase is characterized by ambivalence and by the efforts to defend himself by means of short sleep-regression and childish games in order to get control over the overwhelming emotions or to avoid the coming happenings. During this phase Cyclops is pulled in opposite directions—searching for the security and comfort of old defenses on the one hand while being irresistibly drawn towards becoming an adult on the other hand. In the second phase, a fantasy-dreamlike narrative, Cyclops is in the cave, behaving as if he is a mature, sexualized adult. "On the fourth day Cyclops ran peacefully in the fields hopping from side to side, and climbed the tree and hid among the branches and the leaves of the tree. Only his scared, wondering face could just be discerned among the branches and the leaves of the tree." When Cyclops realizes the size and color of the eye he is described as a "proud Cyclops" but after the masturbation his face, "just discerned among the branches and the leaves of the tree," is described as "scared, wondering." The feelings of pride and elation are thus disturbed by first intuitions of danger and threat, of eroded defenses and the rise of anxiety.

The eye, up to now in a realm under Cyclops' domination, has become nearly autonomous, possessing its own needs, able to act on its own initiative, and threatening to take control of the whole of Cyclops. As Laufer and Laufer (1984) put it, the body, "which until puberty, was experienced as a passive carrier of needs and wishes, now becomes the active force in sexual and aggressive fantasy and behavior" (p. 5). Cyclops can no longer be the plump, loveable creature he had been. He is confused and embarrassed, worried by what he thinks he has to do, but not knowing whether he can succeed and what the consequences of his act would be. He is no longer a child and not yet an adult. He was described as "formed wonderfully well with … stretched neck and straight chin jutting out diagonally upwards"; but now, "sturdy" though he is, "His hair was shorn right down to the roots." Nature, which once was so good to him, is felt still as close to him and loved, but also as alienated and as an object of his aggressiveness.

His mood changes rapidly. After gobbling up "all the leaves, leaving the branches bare" (a manifestation of bodily instinct), Cyclops goes to play a childish game: "He blew soap bubbles, slowly, from a hollow tube. Bubbles completely round, smooth and light, floating. Bubbles fracturing the light into colors.... Cyclops stared a long time at the sun. He felt its heat, and wanted to grab it, and to put it on his tongue." By blowing soap bubbles, he tries to prevent the inevitable and to return to being a child.

But the hopeless pursuit of a lost childhood—although it provides a short comfort in the feeling of being close to the sun again—also increases his pain, frustration, and despair. As these increase he seeks solace in Mother Earth. "He plummeted to the earth like a mast stricken and sinking. His arms were spread out to the side but the front of his body was hard and the earth trembled. Cyclops sank his colored nails into the earth. He pushed and shoved. He dug, and barked angry barks and thrust his head into the earth. The earth was warm. He lay thus many years." Cyclops finds in the earth a temporary refuge. Regression is still possible, and desirable for him—it provides him with a respite to regain his strength. But sleeping or regression do not stop the bodily maturation. And when he awakes from his long sleep he is reborn to feelings and emotions he has never felt before—enslaved by his body's demands (Laufer and Laufer, 1984); first by his huge hunger—he "fell upon the patches of thick green grass and ate them. He opened his mouth and his white teeth chewed the earth. He munched lumps of soil and crushed the stones that wrestled with his white teeth. Behind the thigh of the mountain he saw a lit up green expanse and ran, hopping trampling and kicking over the deep holes, assailing the grasses and the thorns, his mouth biting with hasty, sudden movements."

Like masturbation, the extensive hunger and the voracious eating are new modes of feeling the body. This is not the eating of a child, this is the savage eating of an adolescent monster, eating that aims to assuage the hunger of the developing body, an eating which entails control of the external world. Yet he still eats only grass and this eating does not satisfy him. His eating may seem a mature expression of bodily satisfaction, an acceptance of the new Cyclops, the adult he has become. But it is not a true acceptance. It is not the acceptance of one who is happy with the new function he must fulfill, rather it is "a flight" a defense by displacement of libido (A. Freud, 1958). It is the bitter acceptance of one who surrenders to the knowledge that he has no alternative, one who feels he has become adult, willy nilly, while he is still afraid and angry, and still caught in the toils of the struggle within.

With a sigh Cyclops tries to calm himself again, this time through the recital of a nursery song. Composing the nonsensical song of childhood, he hopes to gain some control of his feelings, or to return to childhood tranquility. Like blowing soap bubbles, singing the song is also part of childhood and its games, which served in the past as a means of diverting and calming himself. Cyclops recurs to them now, since he has no new methods, but they do not help him to cope with the severity of the current anxiety. After singing a few lines his mouth produces "all kinds of whistles, and grunts and snorts and roars" the voice of the unruly unconscious. The children's song, which seems quite innocent and arbitrary, in fact reveals the unconscious, for it contains three significant allusions, two of them ominous. The first allusion is to The Wizard of Oz, a story of the transition from childhood to adulthood, and of the successful search for and formation of identity. But the second is an allusion to the first sentence of Job*: "There was a man in the land of Uz" and brings therefore with it a sense of approaching testing and disaster. The last sentence of the song "And he was called Utzly Gutzly" is an allusion to the Brothers Grimm's story, Rumpelstiltskin. "Rumpelstiltskin" becomes "Utzly Gutzly" in the well-known Hebrew translation of the tale by Abraham Shlonsky. The word play in Hebrew hinges upon the meaning of *utzly* or "give me advice" and the word *gutz* or "midget," a reference to the size of the short man Rumpelstiltskin. In Rumpelstiltskin the usual convention of love fables is reversed. In this story the fulfillment of love is conditional upon the hiding, not revealing, of the lover's identity. The hiding of his identity is the secret of his strength. When his identity is revealed, his relationship with the miller's daughter and the potential relationship with her child end and he must die. Is this not also what the Cyclops fears the future holds for him? Finding his identity, he will meet disaster. As Harry Rand (2000) beautifully shows, Rumpelstiltskin is one of the Grimms' most interesting and complex tales. Rand's reading of the story is confirmatory of this interpretation: Rumpelstiltskin, he finds, is a symbol of male impotence, a failed penis. Cyclops, while trying, through singing the song, to conceal or relieve the emotional stress he is undergoing, actually reveals the intertwined roots of his unconscious fear. He is afraid of realizing his sexual identity lest he lose the infantile, oedipal object of love, and consequently finds himself impotent. The oedipal trap caught in this fantasy situation will be elaborated in the sequel.

Hearing the song he himself created brings Cyclops's unconscious fantasy to life. When he finishes the song, he understands suddenly what is happening to him. "He sang the song again and emitted a hoarse joyful shout: There was a man from the land of Oz toodly pim pam pom, until his voice broke and became a thin screech, and then he got up and looked around threateningly and in dread."

Primal scene, masturbation fantasy, and castration fear

After being overwhelmed by the discovery of his sexual body, the onset of a huge hunger, aggressive and sexual fantasies, and the weaknesses of defenses, Cyclops finds himself in the cave. Singing his song has let him down. Nature, which once defended him, has become threatening, dangerous, boding ill. From within the threat and the fear, the dread and the sense of impotence in the face of a world

---

* In Hebrew the same name—Utz—is used for the land of Job and of The Wizard (which is called in Hebrew The Wizard of Utz).

and his own body which are suddenly hostile to him, he finds himself in the cave, with all his senses alert, and voracious—"the song had increased his hunger." Following the initial separation from his childish self, expressed by his symbolic sleep-death, he is reborn, a different Cyclops, at the cave where he will complete the transition from child to adult. The enclosed space of the cave is at once grave and womb. This scene is very intense and powerful, dominated by both aggressive and sexual meanings and connotations.

An anthropological perspective would perceive this scene as the fantasy equivalent of a rite of passage (Van Gennep, 1960), which in this story takes the form of a violent and aggressive first sexual act. This is the rite of passage to adulthood, the task Cyclops has to accomplish; and this is the focus and the nexus of his ambivalence, his dread, desire, and anxiety. The eating of the humans can be understood as a primitive symbol of a sexual act in the human world, and as an act of initiation (Freud, 1959b). The cave is a symbol of the liminality (Turner, 1969) which is characteristic of the transition phase of rites of passage: a marginal state of betwixt and between, during which one is neither in possession of one's old identity nor of one's new or future one.

The whole scene, however, has specific connotations related to Swift's satire, *Gulliver's Travels*. The bodily changes and the eroding of defenses, which have made possible the great sensual awakening, come to a climax in the presence of the small humans. Freedman (1984) insightfully analyzes Gulliver's discovery of the Lilliputians as the discovery of his own body, and the threat Gulliver experienced as the threat of this discovery to his ideal self-image. Similarly, the brutish, degraded Yahoos ... "are but externalizations of a subjective condition. Their body features are his, his abhorrence a fear and loathing of his own" (p. 474). Cyclops's aggressiveness towards the small humans thus is a displacement of that directed towards his own body as the result of narcissistic injury. Yet, this scene in Cyclops Polyphemus can also be read as a masturbation fantasy, a fantasy in which Cyclops imagines himself facing the task of the adult Cyclops. Masturbation and masturbation fantasies during adolescence normally function to help integrate regressive fantasies into the effort to achieve genital dominance. The adolescent's oedipal fantasies can be allowed into consciousness, in a disguised form, and are then normally re-repressed (Laufer and Laufer, 1984). The "central masturbation fantasy" (Laufer and Laufer, 1984) is the fantasy that answers to multiple regressive satisfactions and the main sexual identifications, and which is a response to the demand of the body to feel something previously denied. Certain kinds of fantasies, for example fantasies that include shame and self-hatred, may lead to a "developmental breakdown," which manifests in dissociation from one's physically mature body; sudden collapse of oedipal identification; failure of the defenses against oedipal aggression and accompanying fantasies of destruction, incest, and hatred of one's own body (p. 40).

Cyclops gazes a long time at the neat, small humans. He examines them and himself alternately. And from this encounter emerges in him an ancient identity involving strength, size, force, and cruelty—he is the giant Cyclops. "He enjoyed seeing the eyes and the noses and the mouths and the ears and all the details of their tiny bodies. He enjoyed seeing their shapely delicate bodies. He yelled with delight when he discovered their miniature genitals. Suddenly his hand whipped out and tore off the two sexual organs." Cyclops ceremonially devours his prey, and drinks their blood, taking intense pleasure in the eating of the living flesh and of the genitals "only the heads he didn't like, so he spat out the hairy skulls."* The ceremony is mythological, savage, appalling by any human standard, an experience of power overwhelming in its totality and extremity and felt as something very close, well known ("his ancient thirst"), latent within him from time immemorial and at the same time strange and alien ("he hated earth, its stones and grasses and its grains of sand and its thorny plants").

The connotations of this scene suggest a primal scene fantasy (Freud, 1914). In *The Odyssey* the human beings were eaten in couples, and the version in the story, "He had two trembling warm bodies upon his tongue," represents the dyad in a primal scene. Primal scene fantasies arouse oedipal libido and consequent fear of castration. This overdetermination mirrors the trap in which Cyclops is caught: He is driven at once by oedipal fantasies and by the urge to perform the deed which is demanded of an adult and which is taboo to a still oedipal child.

After eating the humans, "Cyclops Polyphemus lay down full of happiness and slept a misty sleep, his hand stroking and caressing the small, cute humans. His eye was open, and as fine and clear as ever." After the turbulence and the excitement comes lassitude and relaxation. The eating of the human beings has also aroused mixed feelings and emotions—a sense of achievement for accomplishing a feat, a sense of confidence that his eye (the significant organ) had remained whole, but also a sense of alienation, confusion and uncertainty. These last feelings are the expression both of the fact that he is not ready to be severed from his oedipal maternal love object and because the fantasy was experienced as the fulfillment of the forbidden.

And then the terrible happens—the blindness, the castration (Freud, 1914). The ceremony does not end with incorporation but with a developmental breakdown (Laufer and Laufer, 1984) or a still liminal state of defeat and nonentity, loneliness, alienation, and depersonalization. The regressive satisfaction in the fantasy is judged by the superego as being unacceptable. The punitive castration, therefore, is not surprising. It is described very beautifully through two dreams, very similar to each other but not identical. As in dreams the sequence is not clear, since present tense and past tense interchange. In both dreams the human beings punish Cyclops for his deeds by blinding/castrating him. In the first dream they are "grasping, all of them together, the trunk of a tree, swing-

---

* This comment seems to me the only humoristic-cynical comment in the story. Given the intellectual power of the writer, this comment refers to his attitude—of disgust and repulsion—towards this power, and its inferiority in comparison to the power of the body and body feelings.

ing it upwards, approaching at a run and plunging it into his repulsive eye, his beautiful eye." The second dream happens after the act of the plunging of the trunk into the eye is already completed, and Cyclops is now blind. This dream reveals what is only hinted in the first dream, the ridicule of the human beings: "People make dance steps, full of grace. In the air. Their hands wave in the air. They hold their heads high. A faint smile on their faces, mysterious and arrogant. ... They roll about on the ground like thrown away elastic dolls, their hands on their stomachs. Laughter prostrates them. One points to him and the throttled laughter bursts out and swells."

While in the first dream the assault is painful, physical, in the second dream the psychological injury—the humiliation caused by the laughter—is more powerful. Cyclops responds to the physical injury with revengeful anger: "He tore out a lump of rock. Above his head his two hands stretched tight around the piece of rock. He hurled it into the Atlantic Ocean ... his wild scream accompanying the huge cliff cutting through the air in a whistling arc, threatening in the skies of the world, till he heard the sound of cracking wood and the thunder of wreckage and the roar of huge waves." He responds with helplessness, defeat, and depression at the realization of his castrated status: "In the dim light between the trees he sees the figure of a ridiculous giant. The figure stoops forward in great concentration. Its face is pale, its hands harden over the ground. Its legs are bent in the posture of a leap, pressed against the blocks. He awaits a sign. The flexible, supple and tough body seems to freeze, to solidify in its obstinate posture of powerful, withheld threat. Every nerve in his body is ready, his muscles tense and aching. He waits for some sign. Strange creaks are heard from his broken back. His muscles are about to tear. He stops and awaits a sign. At last Cyclops sees the face that is turned to the ground slowly raised, a tormented face, saturated in reproof. Cyclops studies the face with great interest, unable to tear his gaze away from the gaping black hole in the middle of the forehead."

This paragraph, which is the only whole paragraph in the story which is written in the present tense, powerfully catches the impression of the catastrophic events on the Cyclops. He is now able to feel himself a "ridiculous giant." Only through detachment from his body, a kind of depersonalization, of seeing himself somehow from the outside is he able to face "the gaping black hole in the middle of the forehead."

Instead of having "a large eye, the size of the palm ... of a strange green-blue glittering color ... round and big ... a thick eye, prominent upon the forehead ... like a deep glass ball whose color shifted back and forth between dark green and light blue" he has now "a black hole." Instead of being a sexually matured Cyclops, he is now an impotent, female-like, despised, and ridiculed giant.

Cyclops understands that he is no longer a Cyclops among the Cyclopses. He no longer looks like one, he has not fulfilled his Cyclopian expectations. He is a castrated Cyclops, punished for the act that, had he refrained from carrying it out, would have proved him no true Cyclops.

The end of the rite of passage for Cyclops Polyphemus is therefore pain and despair. His return to the earth is equivocal—part suicide, part return to the womb. He is wounded and beaten. And if he, Cyclops, or the author he reflects, were to remain in this state of regression or self-destruction we would have a portrait of an adolescent in breakdown: he has failed to come to terms with sexuality, with his adult role. He did not achieve separation from his oedipal fantasy, and did not achieve a body representation, which includes physically mature genitalia. He is not happy to be maturing and sees no prospect of compensation for the loss of childhood. The rite of passage to adulthood has been depicted as sadomasochistic, appealing, and fearful. He is left in a state painfully intense and total. There is no exit from the cave where the rite of passage to adulthood has been depicted with a spine-chilling blend of horror and fascination. There is no exit and no succor. The narrative of a journey to the ambivalent fantasy of a symbolic womb–grave ends where it ends: in a self burial, and it offers a wealth of authentic and powerful insights into the world of an adolescent.

Summary

The story "Cyclops Polyphemus" is a very powerful example of an adolescent's use of sublimation—at once masking and revealing the anxieties, desires, and ambivalences experienced during the transition between childhood and adulthood. It embodies a paradox—the most chaotic, primary process fantasies are told through a highly organized and shaped aesthetic form. Laufer and Laufer (1984) refer to masturbation fantasies as inefficient when they bring about feelings of shame, worthlessness, and guilt. In *Creative Writers and Day-Dreaming,* Freud (1959a) describes the secretiveness by which adults conceal their daydreams and fantasies, being sure that they are the only ones who experience them and convinced they are wrong to do so. The poet, in contrast, using his personal daydreams in an aesthetic way, "bribes us by the purely formal—that is, aesthetic—yield of pleasure which he offers us in the presentation of his phantasies" (p. 153). The fantasies of the writer of Cyclops Polyphemus did not block him with shame or guilt. Instead they became fruitful material for creativity, while giving us a rare glimpse into the world of adolescence.

References

Blos, P. (1967), The second individuation process of adolescence. *The Psychoanalytic Study of the Child*, 21:162–166. New Haven, CT: Yale University Press.

Erikson, E. H. (1968), *Identity, Youth and Crisis*. New York: Norton.

Fenichel, O. (1953), Scoptophilic instinct and identifications. In *The Collected Papers of Otto Fenichel (First Series)*. New York: Norton, pp. 373–397.

Freedman, W. (1984), The whole scene of this voyage. A primal scene reading of Gulliver's voyage to Brobdingnag. *Psychoanal. Rev.*, 71:553–567.

—————— (1986), Gulliver's voyage to the country of the Houyhnhnms: Adolescence and the resurgence of the instincts. *Internat. Rev. Psycho-Anal.*, 13:473–486.

Freud, A. (1958), Adolescence. *The Psychoanalytic Study of the Child,* 13:255–277. New Haven, CT: Yale University Press.

Freud, S. (1953), Three essays on the theory of sexuality. *Standard Edition,* 7:123–243. London: Hogarth Press. (Original work published 1905)

—————— (1959a), Creative writers and day-dreaming. *Standard Edition,* 9:141–153. London: Hogarth Press. (Original work published 1908[1907])

————-— (1959b), On the sexual theories of children. *Standard Edition,* 9:207–226. London, Hogarth Press. (Original work published 1908)

—————— (1955), From the history of an infantile neurosis. *Standard Edition,* 17:3–122. London: Hogarth Press. (Original work published 1918[1914])

Laufer, M. (1966), Object loss and mourning during adolescence. *Psychoanalytic Study of the Child,* 21:269–293. New Haven, CT: Yale University Press.

Laufer, M. & Laufer, M. E. (1984), *Adolescence and Developmental Breakdown: A Psychoanalytic View.* New Haven: Yale University Press.

Mahler, M. (1975), *The Psychological Birth of the Human Infant.* New York: Basic Books.

Rakoff, V. M. (1993), Creativity and productivity in adolescence. *Adolescent Psychiatry,* 19:46–57. Chicago: University of Chicago Press.

Rand, H. (2000), Who was Rumpelstiltskin? *Internat. J. Psychoanal.,* 81:963–962.

Turner, V. W. (1969), *The Ritual Process, Structure and Anti-Structure.* Chicago: University of Chicago Press.

Van Gennep, A. (1960), *The Rites of Passage.* London: Routledge and K. Paul. (Original work published 1909)

2 Gustav Klimt (1862–1918)

Arrested adolescent development in a revolutionary artist

David Dean Brockman

Abstract

Gustav Klimt led a very productive and creative life in Vienna during the famous fin-de-siècle time. Klimt's work is extraordinarily novel and his gift of depicting in his portraits the inner life of women and their sexuality has no peers. This chapter presents the hypothesis that he failed to master the tasks of young adulthood after suffering several losses and narcissistic injuries, and as a consequence his personality was arrested at the adolescent level. Another important fact is that Klimt did not have the benefit of an analysis that could have helped him through remembering, repetition, and working through his conscious and unconscious conflicts. His developmental arrest is illustrated in his paintings, which reflect preoccupations with the inner life of women, nudity, sex, and life and death issues. His creativity was generated from that area of his personality, uncontaminated by the arrested development.

Introduction

This chapter is a contribution to the study of the personality of the incomparable Secessionist Viennese artist Gustav Klimt (Arvason, 1998; Belli, 1990). This remarkably talented man, whose repeated interest in women was unequaled and boundless, single-handedly created an art form unequaled in the world. Klimt was a central part of the art and sociopolitical climate in Vienna that made so many contributions to the intellectual and cultural life at the turn of the twentieth century. Although very few facts are known about his early life and adolescence, and he was secretive about his personal life, much can be inferred from his work of over two hundred paintings and several thousand drawings. His artistic development reveals much about his arrested personality, and his compulsion to repeat (Freud, 1914b), together with his unconscious conflicts about women. A selection of his paintings reproduced throughout this chapter graphically shows how he regarded women. Drawing on my work on the transition from adolescence to adulthood (Brockman, 2003), I will show how these paintings reveal certain aspects of his personality that are the result of delayed or arrested adolescent development.

What I would like to emphasize here is the fact that he could not learn from repetition in the natural experience of remembering and processing traumatic memories, which is normally a central part of every successful analytic experience (Freud, 1914b). The analytic situation promotes remembering. A successful recollection of memories of traumatic past events, experiences, relationships, and transferences can lead to interpretative interventions and a working through of many old conflicts that are reenacted in the here-and-now transference and transference neurosis. Klimt did not have the advantage of an analysis of his fixations on the anatomy and psychology of his women models or patrons and unfortunately was left to deal alone with his traumatic background as well as his unconscious conflicts about intimate heterosexuality. His personality remained arrested at the adolescent level and did not proceed to young adulthood.

First, I would like to describe some parts of the sociopsychological and intellectual culture of Vienna during Gustav Klimt's lifetime. An extraordinarily unique ferment existed in the intellectual, political, and psychological life of this city, which had a multiethnic culture that was unusual for the rest of Europe. Vienna, the western capital of the Austro-Hungarian Empire, was made up of a polyglot population of Poles, Hungarians, Slavs, and Germans. Its sizeable Jewish population was very eager to assimilate and assume frontline positions in the arts, the professions, politics, the university, and business. As Schorske has described (1981), there were many contrasts within the culture. The contrasts include the provincial versus the intellectual, the literary versus the journalistic, and the business versus the professional. The elite in all these areas were highly educated and excited by the prospect of learning and contributing to something novel and innovative. "The new culture-makers in the city of Freud thus repeatedly defined themselves in terms of a kind of collective oedipal revolt" against the "paternal culture of classical liberalism" (Schorske, 1981, p. 5).

Politically, there was a curious alignment between the educated liberal middle class and the aristocracy. In fact, liberal political philosophy received a wide reception when a portion of the educated middle class (including some parts of the Jewish population) merged with the politically weak emperor to counteract the more powerful Christian Socialist Party. This occurred when the Christian Socialist party, conservative, nationalistic, German, ant-Slav, and anti-Semitic, defeated the Liberal Party. As Uhl has put it, Vienna became "not so much a 'melting pot' as a 'battlefield of nationalistic chauvinisms, ethnic and social opposites, racism of all kinds and anti-Semitism'" (2000, p. 15). The emperor in Vienna was politically weak overall, without a strong power base, and there was yet another imperial court in Budapest. In Eriksonian terms, there was a kind of mass cultural identity crisis encompassing much turmoil, stress, and strain within the sociopolitical and psychological cultures. On the other hand, all these factors which led to cultural turmoil and social disintegration also played a stimulating and vital part in the emergence of much that was new in art (Klimt and the Art Nouveau Secessionists and a little later Schiele [Kallir, 1980]), in music (Strauss and Mahler), in drama (Schnitzler), in literature (Hoffmanstahl), in architecture

(Otto Wagner), in medicine (Semmelweiss), in science (Hemholtz), in philosophy (Wittgenstein), and in psychology (Freud). In Schorske's words (1981), "by the 1890's the heroes were actors, artists, and critics;" "The life of art became a substitute for the life of action.... Art became almost a religion, the source of meaning and the food of the soul... people turned to a cultivation of the soul" (p. 8). Furthermore, all was not well in the sexual life of the young men and women in Vienna. Young men visited brothels to satisfy their sexual cravings, but young women were left to become hysterics (Janik & Toulmin, 1973; Morton, 1980). (I would add here the life of the psyche for many people of all ages was in great neurotic turmoil.) It is here that Freud's theoretical and clinical contributions to the intellectual and cultural life are important, because his magnum opus *The Interpretation of Dreams* was written in the late 1890's and published in 1900. Thus the new century opened with new ideas about a dynamic unconscious, which was the source of the creative and problem-solving functions of mental life, and these ideas led to newer and deeper insights into mental functioning. Freud's method of interpreting the latent content of dreams revealed the source of their content in the dynamic conflict between infantile sexual wishes and the corresponding defensive operations.

Just as Freud's concepts about the role of sexuality in the development of the personality and the vicissitudes of infantile sexuality changed the culture and influenced its aesthetics, Klimt's art had a revolutionary effect on this same culture. It is not certain if Klimt ever met Freud; but Klimt knew Schnitzler, Freud's friend, and he painted the portrait of the woman patient (Baroness Marie Ferstel) who helped Freud get his university professorship, so it is possible they were acquainted with each other. Klimt repeatedly sought a professorship too, but that honor was denied him. Even if they never met, Klimt must have been aware of Freud's ideas. which were widely discussed in the coffee shops, and Klimt must have read the scathing review of Freud's *Interpretation of Dreams* (1953) in the popular press. And Freud likewise must have known about the controversy over the paintings for the Aula (the entry hall of the University), which I will discuss presently.

In the arts, the traditional liberal rationalist culture, which centered on the ultimate authority of reason, came under attack from many sources, including Freud with his emphasis on the function of the unconscious sexual drive in personality development. Early on, the Emperor Franz Joseph, the Empress Elizabeth, and the government supported and granted many commissions to the Secessionists and to Klimt personally, but this support was withdrawn later.

Thus, it happened in this very interesting time of cultural renaissance that a revolutionary art movement took place. It was first called the Secessionist movement and was characterized by the plain style of architecture created by Otto Wagner, for example, one of the buildings on the famous Ringstrasse, which was created when the emperor ordered the removal of the old wall around the city. (Incidentally, Freud liked to walk around it every night.) Gustav Klimt was a close friend and collaborator of Wagner, but Klimt later broke away to form his own unique style of ornamental painting of nudes, landscapes, and portraits of famous rich women.

Not very much is known about Klimt's early life but there are a few biographical facts of note. Klimt was born in 1862, the second son and one of six children to Ernst Sr. and his wife Anna. That the family was Christian may be inferred, since a painting exists that shows the mother wearing a cross necklace. Ernst Sr. was a gold and silver engraver living in Baumgarten, a poor suburb of Vienna. At age fourteen, Gustav entered the arts and crafts school called the Kuntsgewerbeschule rather than the more prestigious Art Academy, because his plan was to become a teacher in order to help support the family. But since he showed so much promising talent, the Director of the School Ferdinand Laufberger and Klimt's teacher Victor Berger persuaded Klimt to remain at the school for nine years instead of the usual two or three. After finishing there, he formed a partnership with his brother, Ernst Jr., and Franz Matsch called the Kunstcompanie. They received commissions to paint works for the Empress Elizabeth's palace, which led to a famous painting depicting the well-known patrons of the old Burgtheater before it was torn down and also some murals for the Kuntshistorisches building.

Frederick Morton in A Nervous Spendor (1979) describes the high-minded literary and social scene in Vienna in 1888-1899, where both Theodor Herzl and Arthur Schnitzler were lionized playwrights. He notes that Klimt in March of that year "shook off the doldrums which set in after completing the Court Theater

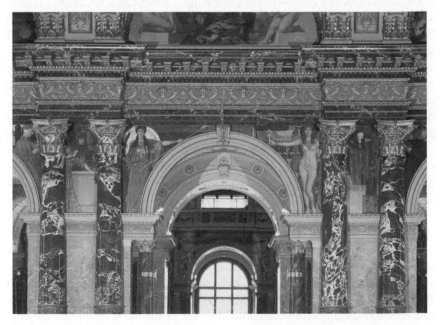

Figure 2.1   "Greek Art" and "Egyptian Art" Fresco, 1890. Erich Lessing, Art Resources, New York.

painting" (p. 308) by long hikes in the Triestestrasse. There, like a rowdy but animal-loving adolescent, he would start a fist-fight with the carriage drivers who abused their horses when they got stuck in the roads muddied from spring rains.

Klimt suffered several major object losses. First, his sister died when he was twelve and then his father, Ernst Sr., died in July 1892 when Gustav was in his thirtieth year, followed by his brother, Ernst, Jr., in December of the same year. The death of his brother left Gustav the guardian of his little niece Helene. Gustav withdrew into a depression. Shortly afterwards, the partnership with the more conservative Matsch dissolved. Klimt's work began to reflect his deep disagreement with his critics. A radical change occurred in his style as he deviated from his originally conservative classicism. For example, his earlier painting of the patrons in the Burgtheater and the Kunsthistorisches stairway panels and ceiling lunettes were classical in the style of Raphael's "School of Athens" painting (Figure 2.1).

The nudes were statuesque and Greek in style and definitely nonerotic. In 1899 Klimt was regarded "the quintessential Austrian" and "the greatest living Austrian painter" (Comini, 1975, p. 7). But now Klimt moved to evolve to a revolutionary style and began painting nudes in more provocative poses: heterosexual, lesbian, and autoerotic.

Klimt's breakup with Matsch was due to differences over how to execute the commission for the Kuntshistorisches building and the most important ceiling paintings for the entry hall (the Aula) of the University to celebrate various departments. Klimt's commission was to paint the panels for the departments of Philosophy, Medicine, and Jurisprudence. His preliminary drawings for the University were not at all what the staid conservative university faculty wanted. Viennese art critics and the entire faculty were appalled by the overt natural nudity with prominently displayed pubic hair. The harshly graphic representation of Life and Death in the Medicine panel (Figure 2.2) was too much for the outraged faculty and they rejected all three works. Even though the faculty eventually approved the work in 1903, after much criticism from the public and the university, Klimt returned the commission of 30,000 crowns. Unfortunately, an air raid fire in World War II destroyed all three paintings. The scathing criticism that he was "depraved" for painting nudes floating in the air severely injured Klimt's prideful self-regard and led to an even greater withdrawal and a deepening of his depression. He expressed his rage in a painting whose title is translated as

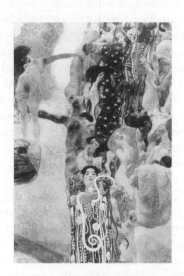

Figure 2.2   Medicine Oil on canvas, 1900–1907.

Goldfish to My Critics (originally *To My Detractors*, 1900–1902), which depicts a leering nude mooning the viewer (Figure 2.3). The woman is mischievously exhibiting her ample bottom and alongside her is a fish head that could suggest Klimt's negative view of his critics and the university faculty.

Klimt was very secretive about his personal life. His most revealing comment was, "Whoever wants to know something about me—as an artist, the only thing—ought to look carefully at my pictures and try to see in them what I am and what I want to do" (Dean, 1996, p. 6). On another occasion he said he was not interested in himself, but in others, "particularly women" (Rogoyska, 1999, p. 3). Comini (1975) suggests an interesting and more intellectual interpretation (but one I think incorrect) that Freud and Klimt were of a similar mind: "For them the interpretation of a symbolic dream, or of a decorative overlay, was the *link* between the conscious and the unconscious life—an interpenetrating link which pointed to the latent content of the psyche or world cycle (p. 6)." My psychoanalytic construction is that Klimt's regression and depressive fixations and preoccupations with sex, sex symbols, couples kissing, and death is that he was a consummate voyeur of the primal scene, women masturbating, and lesbian lovers embracing. He was fascinated with the inner life of women and attempted to capture it on canvas. In fact, in his public life as well, he was a Don Juan–like character who fathered no less than fourteen illegitimate children with his models/mistresses. There is no evidence he had anything to do with his children. Another interesting fact is he pursued Alma Mahler in Venice and probably seduced her there. Alma was "the daughter of a painter and the stepdaughter of fellow Secessionist Carl Moll, who was on intimate terms with Klimt before the turn of the century" (Vergo, 2001, p. 25).

Klimt was unable to form a deep, intimate, monogamous relationship with anyone. He lived with his mother and two sisters. His one platonic relationship with his sister-in-law Emilie Floge (Fischer, 1992), a famous dress designer, was characterized by playful dress-up encounters in his studio garden or on summer vacations rowing on Lake Atter. His daily postcard letters to her when he was away—totaling 400 in all—contained nothing more than banal inanities, such as references to the weather or his hypochondriacal preoccupations about his health. However, he did love cats and kept anywhere from six or more animals at a time in his studio. Often there are animals in his paintings. One of his intellectual interests is that he always carried a copy of Dante's *Divine Comedy* or Goethe's *Faust* in his pocket.

In Peter Vergo's (2001) brilliant essay Between Modernism and Tradition: The Importance of Klimt's Murals and Figure Paintings (pp. 19–39) in the Bailey-edited volume, *Gustav Klimt: Modernism in the Making* (2001), Klimt's three university paintings are interpreted to have been influenced in part by Schopenhauer's philosophic pessimism and by Nietzsche's negative view of science. Schopenhauer wrote of "man's bondage" to an inexorable selfishness as well as to his "Will," something that has governed man's entire life since Adam and Eve (Russell, 1959, p. 25). These influences explain a lot about the pessimistic views

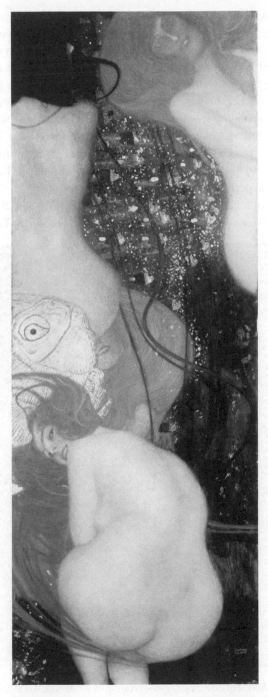

Figure 2.3   Goldfish Oil on canvas, 1901-1902. Scala, Art Resources, New York.

depicted in the Aula ceiling panels, which show Medicine not so much as a healing art, the working of Justice highly questionable, and the depiction of Philosophy as blind except for a woman peering bleakly and despairingly from the depths.

The most well known of Klimt's paintings is *The Kiss* (*Das Kuss,* 1907, figure 2.4), where the man envelopes the kneeling woman in a powerful erotic embrace and kisses her. In this painting from his golden ornamental period, Klimt drew the heterosexual figures first and then covered them over with rich decorations of bright shining gold paint combined with colors of red, blue, and black over a dark brown background and accompanied all over by male and female symbols. Dean (1996) suggests the brightly colored mosaics in Ravenna inspired Klimt during this period.

Many of Klimt's paintings deal with life and death issues, for example *The Three Ages of Woman* (1905), *The Death of Juliet* (1886–1887), and *Sickness,*

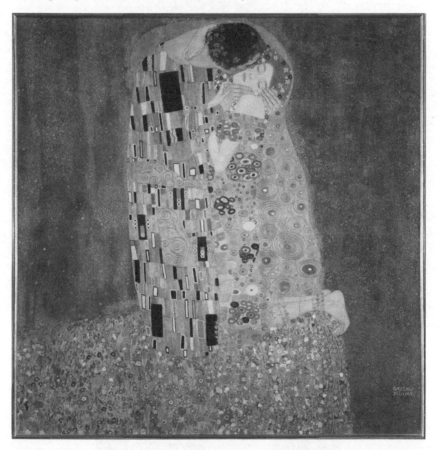

Figure 2.4   The Kiss Oil on canvas, 1907-1908. Erich Lessing, Art Resources, New York.

Mania, and Death above *The Three Gorgons* (1902). *Rita Munk on Her Death Bed* (1912) reminds one of the morbid subject thought patterns in brooding adolescents. In the *Three Ages of Woman* (1905) Klimt has painted a baby girl held by her young mother; standing close by is the old grandmother with sagging skin and gnarled hands and arms. According to Dean (1996) the old woman is based on Auguste Rodin's sculpture of *The Old Courtesan*. Klimt was most provocative in the *Pallas Athena* (1898) painting with its breastplate Medusa sticking out her tongue—a gesture to the critics. It helps to understand the significance of this to know that Athena was the icon of the Secessionists as well as of the Viennese government. A mammoth sculpture of her stood outside the Parliament building, adorned the cupola of the Kuntshistorisches building, and the Viennese people considered themselves the heirs of the Greek Enlightenment. Freud also patted a bust of Athena in his consulting room every morning before he went to work. Alongside Athena's gold plated armor she is holding in her right hand a miniature version of the Nike depicted in *Nude Veritas* (1899, Figure 2.5), a painting in which a nude is holding a mirror facing out to the viewer/critic as if to say, "Who has the dirty mind?" Above her head is Schiller's dictum, "If you cannot please everyone by your actions and your art, please few. It is not good to please the many." In addition, the idea here is clearly the argument that we are seeing the naked truth, which is eternally sexual. The serpent symbolizes sexuality as well as repre-

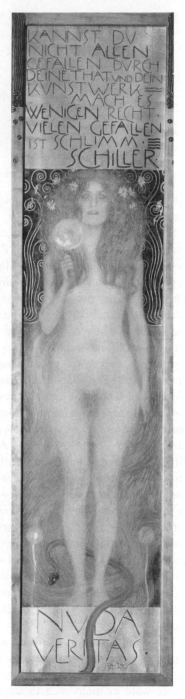

Figure 2.5   Nuda Veritas Oil on canvas, 1899. Erich Lessing, Art Resources, New York.

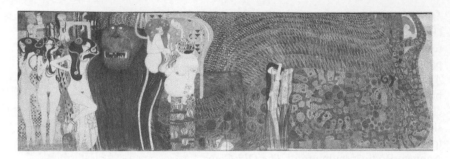

Figure 2.6   Forces of Evil Casein on stucco, 1902. Österreichische Galerie Belvedere.

senting the confrontation with a modern Eve. Truth is symbolized in the mirror in that a reflection can never be false.

Some of Klimt's paintings were meant to be paired and to depict opposites. An example is the Beethoven Frieze (Bouillon, 1987) shown in the fourteenth secessionist exhibition based around Max Klinger's statue of the musician. Depicted here are *The Forces of Evil: Lewdness, Lust, and Excess* (1902, Figure 2.6) and *The Three Gorgons*, which represent disease, madness, and death as well as "debauchery, unchastity, excess, [and] nagging grief" (Dean, 1996, p. 70). Opposing them are *The People Longing for Happiness* and *The Knight*. The latter is reminiscent of the knight in *Life is a Struggle*, who is Klimt himself attempting to overcome evil desires to reach happiness and relief in *Poetry*, which was on the opposite wall. The allegorical meaning here is that the arts are the answer to the baseness of humanity. Dean quotes from the catalogue for the exhibition: "The longing for happiness finds fulfillment in poetry. The arts guide us to the ideal realm where alone we can find joy, pure happiness and pure love." The catalogue also mentioned Schiller's *Ode to Joy*, which was incorporated into Beethoven's Ninth Symphony. In my opinion, all these paintings derive from a serious struggle on Klimt's part to overcome his own misery, the baseness of his sexual desires, and his debauchery. This struggle was to little avail in his life, but was successful in his paintings, where the more noble qualities of his personality and creative gifts could be expressed freely and devoid of conflict. One sees evidence of his creative gift transcending his unconscious conflicts over self-serving sexuality and depressive affects associated with his losses and arrested development in *Hope I* (1903, Figure 2.7). This painting is of his model Herma, who is at least eight months pregnant, and who looks out at the viewer seriously and intently to assert for the moment victory of life over death (represented by a skull above her head).

Klimt returned to the sensual and suspicious theme of powerful women in various media. Women are thus represented as unreliable and sneaky creatures in two paintings titled *Water Serpents I* (1904–1907; 1907, Figure 2.8). There were as many as a thousand drawings, mostly nude, such as *Reclining Nude* (1914–1915) and *Reclining Woman in Lingerie* (1916–1917), that

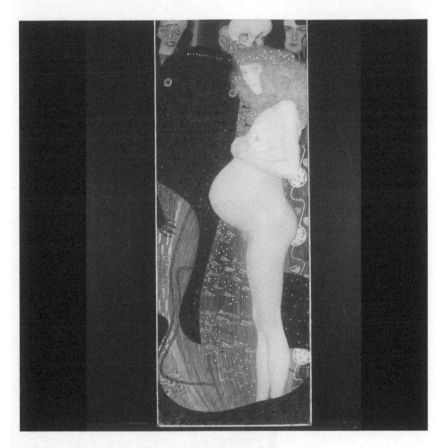

Figure 2.7   Hope I   Oil on canvas, 1903. National Gallery of Canada, Ottawa.

show women masturbating. Another famous painting is of two lesbian women embracing—alongside the couple is a large colorful rooster (Rogoyska, 1999, pp. 102–103).

Despite, or perhaps because of, his notoriety, Klimt gained much success in Vienna through his portraits of women from the aristocratic class and the rich bourgeoisie (Brandstratter, 1974). He unfortunately died too soon at the early age of fifty-six during the 1918 influenza epidemic.

Creativity and psychopathology

In Klimt we see both creativity and significant psychopathology. Freud discusses how the creative artist works in the following passage.

> The motive forces of artists are the same conflicts, which drive other people into neurosis and have encouraged society to construct its institutions.

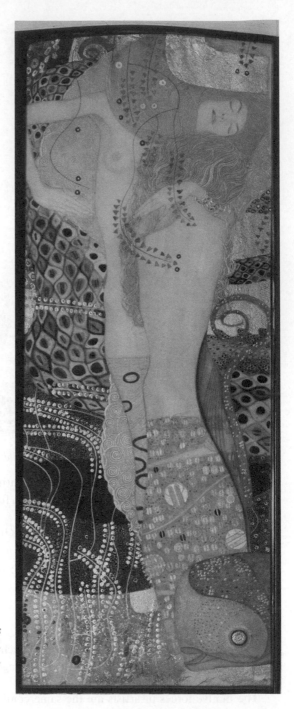

Figure 2.8 Water Serpents I Oil on canvas, 1904-1907. Erich Lessing, Art Resources, New York.

Whence is it that the artist derives his creative capacity is not a question for psychology. The artist's first aim is to set himself free and, by communicating his work to other people suffering from the same arrested desires, he offers them the same liberation. He represents his most personal wishful phantasies as fulfilled; but they only become a work of art when they have undergone a transformation which softens what is offensive in them, conceals their personal origin and, by obeying the laws of beauty, bribes other people with a bonus of pleasure (Freud, 1955, p. 187).

Freud goes on to speculate that the connections between the impressions of the artist's childhood and his life history on the one hand and his works, as reactions to those impressions, on the other is one of the most attractive subjects of analytic examination" (Freud, 1958a, p. 187).

Here Freud is suggesting the process of neutralization or sublimation with which I would heartily agree, but I disagree with the idea that creativity is based on psychopathology. I have suggested that the creativity in young adulthood is not something that is directly connected to psychopathology, but rather is generated from the conflict-free sphere areas of the personality. "The gifted person discovers and realizes his or her potential during the expanding consolidating developmental period from late adolescence on into young adulthood" (Brockman, 2003, p. 246). I also claim that the creative act is consummated in connection with an important personal relationship that facilitates and *crystallizes* a special new way of looking at a part of reality. Klimt probably had many such relationships. The close bond Klimt had with Emile Floge was entirely a platonic internalized relationship that did not reach the level of mature adult heterosexual object relationship in the conventional psychoanalytic sense. In fact, his bond with Emile actually resembled more that of a preadolescent, early adolescent, or late adolescent brother–sister relationship. There were also important artistic influences. Klimt admired and drew inspiration from the impressionist painters and the sculptor Auguste Rodin, whose works he encountered on his many trips to France and Spain. I mentioned earlier the Ravenna mosaics. Finally, the relationships with his mistresses/models were sufficiently intense to provide inspiration, if only of short duration. His curiosity about woman and her sexuality was a constant source of wonder.

Summary

In summary, Gustav Klimt's astonishing work in Vienna during the famous fin-de-siècle time is the result of a productive and creative life shaped by social, cultural, and psychological developmental forces. Klimt's work is extraordinarily novel and his gift of depicting in his portraits the inner life of women and their sexuality has few peers. At the same time, his personality was arrested at the adolescent level. Although his paintings show evidence of his struggles and preoccupations with the inner life of women, nudity, sex, and life and death issues, his creativity itself was generated from that area of his conflict-free personality uncontaminated by the arrested development.

Acknowledgments

The paintings depicted in this chapter are reproduced by the kind permission of the following galleries to which they belong or the owners of the copywrights for their photographs: Erich Lessing, Art Resources, New York (Figures 2.1, 2.4, 2.5, and 2.8), the Oesterreichische Galerie Belvedere (Figure 2.6), Scala Art Resources, New York (Figure 2.3), and the National Gallery of Canada, Ottawa (Figure 2.7).

References

Arnason, H. H. (1998), *History of Modern Art*, Painting, Sculpture, Architecture and Photography, 4th ed. New York: Abrams.

Bailey, C. B. (2001), *Gustav Klimt and Modernism in the Making*. New York: Abrams.

Belli, G. (1990), *Gustav Klimt Masterpieces*. Boston: Little, Brown, & Company.

Bouillon, J. P. (1987), *Klimt: Beethoven The Frieze for the Ninth Symphony,* trans., M. Heron. New York: Skira/Rizzoli.

Brandstatter, C. (1994), *Klimt und der Frauen*. Vienna: Verlaggeesellschaft.

Brockman, D. D. (2003), *From Late Adolescence to Young Adulthood*. Madison, CT: International Universities Press.

Comini, A. (1975), *Gustav Klimt*. New York: George Braziller.

Dean, C. (1996), *Gustav Klimt*. New York: Phaidon Press.

Fischer, W. G. (1992), *Gustav Klimt & Emilie Floge: An Artist and His Muse*. Woodstock, NY: Overlook Press.

Freud, S. (1955), The Interpretation of Dreams, *Standard Edition*, Vol. 4. London: Hogarth Press, 1955. (Originally published in 1900)

_____ (1913), The claims of psychoanalysis to scientific interest, *Standard Edition*, 13:165–190. London: Hogarth Press. 1955.

_____ (1912) On the universal tendency to debasement in the sphere of love, 11:177–190. London: Hogarth Press. 1958.

_____ (1914) Remembering, repeating, and working through. 12:145–156. London: Hogarth Press.1958.

Janik, A. & Toulmin, S. (1973), *Wittgenstein's Vienna*. New York: Simon & Schuster.

Kallir, J. (1980), *Gustav Klimt and Egon Schiele*. New York: Crown Publishers, Inc.

Morton, F. (1979), *A Nervous Splendor: Vienna 1888/1889*. London: Penguin Books.

Rogoyska, J. (1999), *Klimt*. Bonn, Germany: Parkstone Press, Ltd.

Russell, B. (1959), *A History of Western Philosophy*. New York: Simon and Schuster.

Schorske, C. E. (1981), *Fin-de-Siècle Vienna: Politics and Culture*. New York: Vintage Books.

Uhl, H. (2000), Fin-de-siècle Vienna and the ambivalence of modernism. In: *Klimt's Women*, ed. T. G. Natter & G. Frodl. New Haven, CT: Yale University Press, pp. 14–17.

Vergo, P., Between modernism and tradition: The importance of Klimt's murals and figure paintings. In Gustav Klimt: Modernism in the Making, ed. C. B. Bailey. New York: Abrams, pp. 19–39.

Section II

Special section

Difficult challenges—
Creative solutions

3 Saving adolescents

Richard Rosner

Abstract

This chapter is based on the Schonfeld Award presentation at the 2005 Annual Meeting of the American Society for Adolescent Psychiatry, in which Dr. Richard Rosner summarized and synthesized four aspects of his life's work that are relevant to the mission of ASAP, and which are conceptualized as ways of "saving adolescents": 1) education and training in adolescent psychiatry, 2) forensic psychiatry, 3) addiction medicine, and 4) moral philosophy.

The 2005 William A. Schonfeld memorial lecture

Core to the mission of the American Society for Adolescent Psychiatry (ASAP) are the tenets that adolescence is a critical developmental period that carries with it many psychosocial risks, and that treating adolescents effectively requires special knowledge and skills. The William A. Schonfeld Award of ASAP honors the first president of the organization; the award is given to individuals recognized for their outstanding contributions to the field of adolescent psychiatry, as well as for their excellence and dedication to the clinical practice of adolescent psychiatry throughout the course of their career. This chapter is based on the recipient's presentation at the 2005 ASAP Annual Meeting, in which he summarized and synthesized four aspects of his life's work that are relevant to the mission of ASAP, and which are conceptualized as ways of "saving adolescents": (1) education and training in adolescent psychiatry, (2) forensic psychiatry, (3) addiction medicine, and (4) moral philosophy.

Education and training in adolescent psychiatry

For the foreseeable future, there is likely to continue to be a gap between the mental health needs of teenagers and the number of practitioners available to meet those needs. Although there are efforts being made to increase enrollment in American Council on Graduate Medical Education–(ACGME) accredited residency programs in child and adolescent psychiatry, no one expects that those efforts will succeed soon in training sufficient child and adolescent specialists to meet the current and immediately anticipated needs of teenagers in America. Saving adolescents will require that a large number of general psychiatrists take the time to acquire the knowledge and skills needed to help youngsters. ASAP is in the forefront of the effort to attract general psychiatrists to work with teen-agers. ASAP has reorganized itself from being a federation of regional chapters into a unified national structure. The educational programs at our annual conventions provide a convenient route to obtain clinically relevant information about the diagnosis and treatment of adolescent mental disorders. Those general psychiatrists who wish to expand the size and scope of their practice by including adolescents can find in ASAP the continuing medical education courses they need to address this underserved population of potential patients.

ASAP's position on training in adolescent psychiatry has been consistent. Those persons who wish to work with both children and adolescents should be trained in child and adolescent psychiatry. Those persons who wish to work with adolescents and adults should not have to be trained in child and adolescent psychiatry, but should have the option of supplementing their general psychiatry training with additional training in adolescent psychiatry. For example, additional training in adolescent psychiatry can be obtained by taking elective clinical experiences in adolescent psychiatry during the general psychiatry residency. In the past, when ASAP surveyed the ACGME-accredited child and adolescent psychiatry residencies, some of those child and adolescent psychiatry residencies (for example, those that could not fill all of their positions) expressed willingness to offer one year of training in purely adolescent psychiatry. ASAP's Accreditation Council on Fellowships in Adolescent Psychiatry, which I have been involved with since its inception, developed and published criteria to evaluate the quality of the training offered in such one-year adolescent psychiatry residency programs (Rosner, 1997; 2003a; 2003c).

As an alternative pathway to formal residency or fellowship training, after graduation from a general psychiatry residency, additional training in adolescent psychiatry can be obtained by on-the-job training, by continuing medical education courses, and by self-guided systematic independent study. The ASAP-endorsed *Textbook of Adolescent Psychiatry* (Rosner, 2003c) and *Adolescent Psychiatry*, ASAP's annual series of volumes, are useful components of a program of self-guided systematic independent study.

The American Board of Adolescent Psychiatry (ABAP), incorporated as an entirely separate organization from ASAP, serves the important function of distinguishing between (1) those persons who claim to possess the knowledge essential to the care and treatment of adolescents and (2) those persons who have objectively demonstrated that they possess the knowledge essential to the care and treatment of adolescents (by successfully passing ABAP's credentialing and examination processes).

Initially intended as a demonstration project, the New York Chapter of ASAP cooperated with ASAP's Accreditation Council on Fellowships in Adolescent Psychiatry to develop a one-semester training program, accredited for 25–1/2 hours of continuing medical education, for general and forensic psychiatrists who sought additional knowledge about adolescents and adolescent psychiatry. The course has subsequently been integrated into the forensic psychiatry residency programs offered at New York University Medical Center, New York Medical College, Albert Einstein College of Medicine of Yeshiva University, and the medical schools of Columbia and Cornell. The course has functioned as a model of how to integrate training in adolescent psychiatry into the curriculum of other psychiatric residency programs, without having to create freestanding residency programs in adolescent psychiatry per se. Graduates of the course have become members of ASAP, have been certified by the American Board of Adolescent Psychiatry, and have become elected officers of both ASAP's New York Chapter and ASAP's national organization.

Forensic psychiatry

The March 1, 2005, decision of the United States Supreme Court in the case of Roper versus Simmons is a dramatic demonstration of saving adolescents through the interface of adolescent psychiatry and forensic psychiatry. In that case, the Court ruled that the U.S. Constitution prohibits the execution of a juvenile who was under 18 when the crime was committed. The American Society for Adolescent Psychiatry was in the lead among the various medical amici curiae that submitted legal briefs to the U.S. Supreme Court against the death penalty for adolescents in the Roper case. However, there are myriad opportunities in smaller, local, and individual legal cases where adolescent psychiatrists can create alliances with general and forensic psychiatrists and with attorneys to work together in saving adolescents.

From a public health standpoint, it is a curious fact that the city, state, and federal governments have no affirmative obligation to evaluate the mental health of teenagers at large in the community. However, the moment that a teenager is taken into custody by the police and held in detention, there is a governmental obligation to evaluate the mental condition of that teenager and to provide appropriate mental health care and treatment. In this manner, many youngsters who would otherwise never obtain a mental health evaluation are identified as in need of mental health (including substance abuse) services. Thus the juvenile justice system has become a de facto mental health system (Farmer et al., 2003). (This is true of the criminal justice system in general. See Lamb and Weinberger, 1998.) Unfortunately, the majority of general and forensic psychiatrists who work in the juvenile justice and adult correctional systems lack the knowledge and skills needed to evaluate and treat teenagers. Furthermore, in many instances there is a lack of continuity of care so that adolescents who are identified as in need of mental health services while in detention are not routinely and effectively referred to community-based mental health services upon their release from detention. Saving adolescents in detention, and promoting their post-detention care and treatment, will require an active alliance between the general and forensic psychiatrists who work in correctional and community-based settings and the adolescent psychiatrists who have the knowledge and skills needed to treat teenagers.

Even for adolescents who are not held in detention, there are opportunities for adolescent psychiatrists to cooperate with attorneys and forensic psychiatrists in saving adolescents. For example, when a juvenile is arrested the law requires that the police read the Miranda rights (the right to remain silent, the right to refuse to answer questions, and the right to be represented by an attorney) to him or her. But teenagers are vulnerable to witting and unwitting influence by the police that may undermine their ability to understand and assert their Miranda rights. Some adolescents who confess to criminal acts, who do not exercise their right to remain silent, who do not demand that an attorney be provided for them, may be incompetent to have waived their Miranda rights. Adolescent psychiatrists working with attorneys and forensic psychiatrists have a role to play in the evaluation of whether or not a particular adolescent was competent to have waived his or her Miranda rights, including whether or not a particular adolescent was competent to confess to a criminal act. In general, it is the obligation of a defendant in a criminal case to assert that he or she was not competent to have waived his or her Miranda rights. Not all attorneys and not all forensic psychiatrists know that teenagers may respond to being informed of their Miranda rights differently from adults. *Voluntariness* is the key legal criterion in determining whether or not a person's waiver of Miranda rights was valid. Teenagers may hear that they have the right to refuse to answer questions from the police and prosecutors, but may not understand or believe or be able to apply what they have heard to their own immediate reality. Teenagers may be unable to reconcile being told that they do not have to answer questions, on the one hand, and then being asked questions, on the other hand. One role of an adolescent psychiatrist is to bring these matters to the attention of attorneys or forensic psychiatrists, to raise the issue of a teenager's possible incompetence to have waived his or her Miranda rights.

Similarly, at a later stage of the criminal justice system's processes, a defendant may be examined to determine his or her competence to stand trial. That is, whether or not he or she "has sufficient present ability to consult with his lawyer with a reasonable degree of rational understanding—and whether he has a rational as well as a factual understanding of the proceedings against him" as set forth by the U.S. Supreme Court in the case of *Dusky v. United States* (1960). Attorneys and forensic psychiatrists, who are used to adult clients, may have difficulty communicating with teenagers, let alone evaluating their competence to stand trial. Teenagers may be unable to understand and apply abstract legal principles to the specifics of their own legal case. For example, that even if they have engaged in a criminal act, they are entitled to an attorney to represent them and defend them against the legal charges. An adolescent psychiatrist can *translate* communications between attorneys and their adolescent clients, to make sure that the words that are spoken by the attorney are genuinely understood by the adolescent defendant. The adolescent psychiatrist can discern that the teenager has only a factual, but not a rational, understanding of the proceedings again him or her, thus, that the teenager is not competent to stand trial.

While it is uncommon for a defense attorney to assert that a client is not criminally responsible due to mental disease or mental defect, at times it may be the only defense that is feasible. In many states, the defense of "not guilty by reason of insanity" is based on the American Law Institute's 1955 criteria: "A person is not responsible for criminal conduct if at the time of such conduct as a result of mental disease or mental defect he lacks substantial capacity either to appreciate the criminality of his conduct or to conform his conduct to the requirements of law" (American Law Institute, 2003). There is some question as to whether or not adolescents generally (as compared to adults) have an impairment of their capacity to appreciate their conduct. Similarly, there is some question as to whether or not adolescents generally (as compared to adults) have an impairment of their capacity to conform their conduct to the requirements of law. By bringing to the attention of attorneys and forensic psychiatrists that a teenager may have known what he was doing, but may not have appreciated what he was doing, adolescent psychiatrists can make important contributions to saving adolescents within the juvenile and adult criminal justice systems.

Whether the issue is competence to waive Miranda rights, competence to stand trial, or insanity as a defense against criminal charges, saving adolescents may constitute excluding teenagers from inappropriate punishment, and diverting adolescents from the criminal justice system to the mental health system. Towards the end of saving adolescents caught up in the criminal justice system by facilitating constructive alliances with attorneys and forensic psychiatrists, ASAP has established liaisons with the American Academy of Forensic Sciences (AAFS) and the American Academy of Psychiatry and the Law (AAPL).

Addiction medicine

Many of the teenagers who come to the attention of the criminal justice system are caught in the snare of substance abuse. While it is true that attorneys and forensic psychiatrists have much to learn from adolescent psychiatrists, it is equally true that adolescent psychiatrists have much to learn from specialists in addiction medicine and addiction psychiatry. By the time they have graduated from high school, the majority of teenagers have used an illegal substance. We are currently unable to predict reliably which youngsters will, and which will not, spontaneously and successfully resist the forces that lead from substance use to substance abuse to substance dependence. We are obliged to consider all teenagers as at risk for drug addiction and to develop our skills in the diagnosis and treatment of adolescents addicted to both legal and illegal drugs (Rosner, 2005). The public health risk of addiction to legal drugs needs to be stressed: more people will die from the effects of tobacco and alcohol than from the effects of all illegal drugs combined. ASAP's Task Force on Adolescent Addiction recently presented a major educational program to teach the essentials of addiction psychiatry to adolescent psychiatrists. Part of the contents of that program were published in Volume 29 of ASAP's annual series, *Adolescent Psychiatry.*

There are many reasons why substance use, abuse, and dependence are so common among teenagers. We live in a society that is metaphorically *addicted* to immediate gratification, turning for instant satisfaction to television, to computers, and to overconsumption of material goods. Apart from organized religion, what vision do we offer our youngsters as a counterweight to self-indulgent materialism? The success of programs based on spiritual values, such as Alcoholics Anonymous, is illustrative of the help these values offer in breaking free of addiction.

The Twelve-Step self-help model of Alcoholics Anonymous (AA) is the most widely available treatment for substance abusers. The separate self-help organizations modeled on AA include Narcotics Anonymous, Cocaine Anonymous, Marijuana Anonymous, Over-Eaters Anonymous, Gamblers Anonymous, and Survivors-of-Incest Anonymous. AA is a fellowship that offers a spiritual (rather than a religious) vision of the good life. The U. S. government's report on Project Match, a research study under the auspices of the National Institute of Alcoholism and Alcohol Abuse (NIAAA), demonstrated that AA's style of Twelve-Step Facilitation Therapy works as well as cognitive-behavioral therapy or motivational enhancement therapy (the latter is based on motivational interviewing) (Project MATCH Research Group, 1993; 1998). AA helps substance abusers make the transition from self-destructive immediate gratification to societal-enhancing delayed-gratification. AA gives its participants a vision of a life that is worth living; it is inspirational. As adolescent psychiatrists, we need to learn how to use the inspirational power of AA's spiritual fellowship to complement our scientific treatments to foster the growth and development of our patients. The idealism of youth, a feature of normal development, can be a powerful force for good.

Many psychiatrists have distrusted the AA approach and seen it as antagonistic. What makes some of our colleagues uncomfortable with Alcoholics Anonymous is the very spirituality that is AA's strength. Perhaps we need to disentangle spirituality from religion, from mythology, from fairy tales. The word *spirituality* sounds uncomfortably similar to *spirits* and *sprites*. Words that sound similar do not necessarily refer to similar things. Spirituality is not about ghosts, angels, and demons. In secular terms, spirituality is about values. There is an initial and superficial resemblance between ghosts and values, neither of them is visible, neither of them is material, neither of them exists in the same way that a car or a house or a chocolate bar exists; but that is the end of the resemblances. The spiritual vision Alcoholics Anonymous advances is set forth in the Twelve Steps of AA. The Twelve Steps are shown in Table 3.1.

Bowen and MacDougall (2001) have noted that each of these steps corresponds to a specific value which, although not explicitly stated, is nonetheless fundamental. The values associated with each step are summarized in Table 3.1.

Twelve-Step self-help groups like AA are ubiquitous, free, and effective for many adolescent substance abusers. In order to make intelligent referrals to these therapeutic resources, all adolescent psychiatrists who work with teenagers should

Table 3.1   AA Twelve Steps and Corresponding Values

Step	Statement[a]	Value[b]
I	"We admitted we were powerless over alcohol[c] and our lives had become unmanageable."	Honesty
II	"We came to believe that a Power greater than ourselves could restore us to sanity."	Hope
III	"We made a decision to turn our will and our lives over to the care of God as we understood Him."	Faith
IV	"We made a searching and fearless moral inventory of ourselves."	Courage
V	"We admitted to God, to ourselves, and to another human being that exact nature of our wrongs."	Integrity
VI	"We became entirely ready to have God remove all these defects of character."	Willingness
VII	"We humbly asked Him to remove our shortcomings."	Humility
VIII	"We made a list of all persons we had harmed, and became willing to make amends to them all."	Compassion
IX	"We made direct amends to such people wherever possible, except when to do so would injure them or others."	Justice
X	"We continued to take personal inventory, and when we were wrong promptly admitted it."	Perseverance
XI	"We sought through prayer and meditation to improve our conscious contact with God, as we understand Him, praying only for knowledge of God's will for us and the power to carry that out."	Spiritual Awareness
XII	"Having had a spiritual awakening as the result of these steps, we tried to carry this message to alcoholics,[d] and to practice these principles in all our affairs."	Service

[a] Used with permission from AA (See acknowledgement at end of chapter).
[b] From Bowen and White, 2001.
[c] Narcotics Anonymous says "powerless over addiction," Gamblers Anonymous says "powerless over gambling."
[d] Narcotics Anonymous says "addicts."

be familiar with the 12 Steps and with the specific values to which each step corresponds. When dealing with some teenagers, it is more effective to focus on the specific value associated with the step being considered. With other teenagers, it may be more effective to ask what relevant meaning the adolescent can find from his or her personal interpretation of the language of the step.

There are 12-Step groups for agnostics, for atheists, and for secular humanists. The language of the 12 Steps is meant to be inclusive, for example, the phrases "God as we understand Him" and "a power greater than ourselves" can refer to Nature, the cosmos, or any entity/concept that is not one's self, that is not as limited as one's self, and with which one can have a personal relationship. (The Jewish existentialist, Martin Buber, wrote movingly about having a personal encounter with a tree.)

Moral philosophy

We live in a time of anti-intellectualism, moral relativism and *political correctness* which makes many of us reluctant to assert and advocate for the values to which we adhere. However, we should not mistake every person's equal right to state his or her opinion, on the one hand, with every person's opinion being of equal worth, on the other hand. Those opinions that can be supported by facts and reasoned arguments are superior to those opinions that are not supported by facts and reasoned arguments (Rosner 1996, Rosner and Weinstock, 1990).

Adolescents need moral guidelines. We must not abandon our adolescents to a wasteland, to the equally unacceptable poles of immoral materialism and irrational religion. We need to offer them a moral framework derived from sound principles and grounded on shared values. What are the values that we stand for? In so far as we are citizens of the United States of America, we are advocates of legal equality (all persons are equal before the Law), and we are advocates of human rights (no one may be deprived of life, liberty, or property except by due process of law). In so far as we are scientists, we are advocates of truth, honesty, and rationality. In so far as we are physicians, based upon the traditions of medicine, we are advocates of nonmalificence (do no harm) and of benevolence (do good). In so far as we are adolescent psychiatrists, we are advocates of respect for persons (including those impaired by mental disorders) and of fostering healthy human growth. In our commitment to our shared values, we should not be reticent in offering ourselves as models for potential emulation by our patients.

Moral relativism undermines our confidence in our shared moral values. We are told that each culture determines its own morality; that there is no way to determine moral right and wrong outside of a specific cultural framework. In contrast, however, no one would say that each culture determines its own science; that there is no way to determine science outside of a specific cultural framework. If one culture said that the earth was round, and another culture said that the earth was flat, no one would accept that each culture was equally correct. Rather, we would insist that the different scientific assertions be tested to establish which was right and which was wrong. We use scientific techniques to test scientific assertions of facts. Some, but not all, scientific assertions can be tested by current scientific techniques. (Who can currently test whether anything existed before The Big Bang? Who can currently test whether or not String Theory is correct?) We hope science will advance so that, in the future, our scientific techniques will be able to test scientific assertions that cannot now be tested. The same line of thinking applies to the evaluation of disagreements about morality as applies to the evaluation of disagreements about science. We should test moral assertions as rigorously as we test scientific assertions. We use philosophic techniques to test moral assertions. Necessarily, the techniques of philosophy are different from the techniques of science. Some, but not all, moral assertions can be tested by current philosophic techniques. We hope philosophy will advance so that, in the future, our philosophic techniques will be able to test moral assertions that cannot now be tested (Rachels, 2003).

A literal belief in revealed truth as set forth in sacred texts (the Bible or the Koran, for example), common in adherents to fundamentalist religions, also undermines our confidence in our shared moral values. This kind of narrow view holds that whatever God commands as set forth in the sacred text is good, and that whatever God forbids is bad. However, it is reasonable to ask, as a moral philosopher might: "Is what God commands good because God commands it; or is God commanding it because it is good?" This is a subtle but crucial distinction. If God commands us to do something because God knows that it is good because of sound moral principles and moral reasons, then it is not God's command that makes it good. If what makes something good is that God commands us to do it, it follows that if God told us to do the exact opposite thing, then that opposite thing would (by definition) be good.

Thus, either God is arbitrary (anything God commands is good, and its opposite would be good if God commanded us to do its opposite) or God has commanded us to do things that are good because of moral principles and moral reasons that are independent of God's commands. For most religious people, it is unacceptable that God is arbitrary. They share an interest in determining sound moral principles and sound moral reasoning with adherents to secular philosophy (Rachels, 2003).

There have been many attempts to provide an objective, rational grounding for moral principles and moral reasoning. If adolescent psychiatrists are to save adolescents from America's current moral wasteland, the psychiatrists must have a basic understanding of the two leading philosophical theories of moral justification.

The first of these theories essentially says that the end justifies the means—what makes an action good is that its results are good. The most famous advocates of this position are the Englishmen Jeremy Bentham and John Stuart Mill.* As an initial introduction to moral reasoning, Bentham and Mill offer guidelines about what kinds of action one should pursue. They suggest that, given the choice between a variety of actions, one should always choose the action that leads to the greatest good for the greatest number of persons. Teaching adolescents to consider the long-term (as well as short-term) consequences of their potential actions is important. Teaching adolescents to consider the consequences of their potential actions on other people (as well as on themselves) is important. Bentham and Mill would have us teach adolescents to choose the course of action that produces the best long-term and short-term consequences for others and for themselves (Rachels, 2003).

---

* For a fuller discussion of the views of these philosophers, see Rachels's *Elements of Moral Philosophy* (2003).

The second of these theories says that no one should do any action that he or she would not want any other similarly situated person to do in the same circumstances, that we should live according to universal rules that apply to all persons equally at all times. This position holds that the autonomy of all persons should be respected, that no person should be used merely as a means to someone else's ends. The most famous advocate of this position is the German Immanuel Kant. As an initial introduction to moral reasoning, Kant offers guidelines about what kinds of action should be avoided. It is important to teach adolescents that (absent a morally relevant difference) that what is permitted for oneself should be permitted for everyone, that no one is entitled to rights and privileges that he or she would not accord to all people. It is important to teach adolescents that people should not be manipulated, exploited, or used to attain whatever ends the adolescent is seeking, that all people should be respected (Rachels, 2003).

Conclusion

Saving adolescents is not easy. Given the gap between the numbers of teenagers in need of services and the paucity of mental health personnel trained to address that need, it will be necessary to encourage general psychiatrists to obtain the knowledge and skills required to work effectively with youth. It is appropriate for adolescent psychiatrists to focus on high-risk groups—those in juvenile justice settings, and substance abusers. It will be necessary to work with forensic psychiatrists and attorneys to use the justice system to reach troubled teenagers who would not usually seek mental health services on their own initiative. It will be necessary to work with specialists in addictions to learn how to diagnose and treat adolescents who suffer from comorbid illnesses such as mental disorders and substance abuse. It will be necessary to oppose materialism, relativism, and unintelligent religious authoritarianism. It will be necessary to teach sound moral principles, grounded in sound moral justification, to offer an alternative to blind self-indulgence and willful selfishness. We should not be reluctant to affirm our shared values. Who we are, and what we are, the models we offer of responsible, rational commitment to human well being, may be our most important asset in our goal of saving adolescents.

Acknowledgments

Dr. Rosner was founding president of the Accreditation Council on Fellowships in Adolescent Psychiatry (ACFAP), a semiautonomous component of ASAP. During his tenure, ACFAP developed and published the Standards for Fellowships in Adolescent Psychiatry (Rosner, 1997). The ASAP-endorsed *Textbook of Adolescent Psychiatry* initially was proposed by ACFAP as an ASAP project (Rosner, 2003c).

Dr. Rosner participated in 24 graduate school courses in the departments of philosophy at New York University and Columbia University, with a concentration in ethics. Dr. Rosner edited two editions of the book *Principles and Practice of Forensic Psychiatry* (1994; 2003b) and co-edited the book *Ethical Practice in Psychiatry and the Law* (Rosner and Weinstock, 1990).

The American Society of Addiction Medicine certified Dr. Rosner in addiction medicine in 2004. During his tenure as president of ASAP, he created ASAP's Task Force on Adolescent Addiction, arranged that approximately one-third of scientific program at ASAP's annual convention was focused on adolescent addiction, and facilitated the publication of much of that portion of the program in Volume 29 of *Adolescent Psychiatry*.

The Twelve Steps are reprinted with permission of Alcoholics Anonymous World Services, Inc. (A.A.W.S.). Permission to reprint the Twelve Steps does not mean that A.A.W.S. has reviewed or approved the contents of this publication, or that A.A,W.S. necessarily agrees with the views expressed herein. AA is a program of recovery from alcoholism *only*—use of the Twelve Steps in connection with programs and activities which are patterned after AA, but which address other problems, or in any other non-AA context, does not imply otherwise. Additionally, while AA is a spiritual program, AA is not a religious program. Thus, AA is not affiliated or allied with any sect, denomination, or specific religious belief.

References

American Law Institute (2003), Model Penal Code, 1955. In *Principles and Practice of Forensic Psychiatry*, 2nd ed., ed. R. Rosner. London: Edward Arnold, p. 214.

Bowen, F. W., & MacDougall, J. A. (2001), *Clinician's Guide to Spirituality*. New York: McGraw Hill.

Farmer, E. M., Burns, B. J., Phillips, S. D., Angold, A., & Costello, E. J. (2003), Pathways into and through mental health services for children and adolescents. *Psychiatr. Serv.*, 54:60–66.

Lamb, H. R. & Weinberger, L. E. (1998), Persons with severe mental illness in jails and prisons: A review. *Psychiatr. Serv.*, 49:1094–1095.

Project MATCH Research Group (1993), Project MATCH (Matching Alcoholism Treatment to Client Heterogeneity): Rationale and methods for a multisite clinical trial matching patients to alcoholism treatment. *Alcohol Clin. Exp. Res.*, 17:1130–1145.

_____ (1998), Matching alcoholism treatments to client heterogeneity: Project MATCH three-year drinking outcomes. *Alcohol Clin. Exp. Res.*, 22:1300–1311.

Rachels, J. (2003), *The Elements of Moral Philosophy*. New York: McGraw-Hill.

Rosner, R. (1994), *Principles and Practice of Forensic Psychiatry*. London: Chapman & Hall.

_____ (1996), Ethical practice in the forensic sciences and justification of ethical codes, *J. Forensic Sci.*, 41:913–915.

_____ (1997), Report of the Accreditation Council on Fellowships in Adolescent Psychiatry. *Adolescent Psychiatry*, 21:389–407. Hillsboro, NJ: The Analytic Press.

_____ (2003a), Education and training in adolescent psychiatry. In *Textbook of Adolescent Psychiatry*, ed. R. Rosner. London: Edward Arnold.

_____ ed. (2003b), *Principles and Practice of Forensic Psychiatry*, 2nd ed. London: Edward Arnold.

_____ ed. (2003c), *Textbook of Adolescent Psychiatry*. London: Edward Arnold.
_____ (2005) The scourge of addiction: What the adolescent psychiatrist needs to know, *Adolescent Psychiatry*, 29:19–31. Hillsboro, NJ: The Analytic Press.
_____ & Weinstock, R., eds. (1990), *Ethical Practice in Psychiatry and the Law*. New York: Plenum.

4   Toward a better juvenile justice system[*]

A city-state partnership

Johnny L. Williamson, Carl C. Bell, R. Gregg Dwyer, and Richard L. Frierson

Abstract

The care and protection of juvenile offenders are the responsibilities of child welfare agencies, education systems, social services, law enforcement, family courts, juvenile correctional facilities, and mental health providers. How can these entities function together? What information can be used and shared to benefit children, and what potential risks exist? This paper addresses these questions from a broad systems approach to specific examples, beginning with an overview of the magnitude of mental health issues among incarcerated youth. A description of a city-state partnership program based on community psychiatry principles is provided.

Introduction

As the field of psychiatry moves into the 21st century, it will become increasingly possible to take advantage of the science discovered during the 1990 National Mental Health Institute's decade of the brain. Accordingly, we will be in a position to use our understanding of behavioral genetics and the various normal and psychopathologic mechanisms occurring within the brain. Already, research suggests that we can accurately identify children who are at extremely high risk for developing schizophrenia as early as ages 8–10, and there is some evidence that by treating such children with prophylactic medication we can prevent them from becoming clinically ill (McFarlane, 2001). Family-based approaches to prevention, which reduce risk factors and increase protective factors for early adolescents, are efficacious interventions for the prevention of disorders like depression (Beardslee, Gladstone, Wright, and Cooper, 2003) and prevention of HIV risk behaviors (Bhana et al., 2004). Further, the biology of resilience is becoming known and interventions will soon be developed from this new science (Charney, 2004). In addition to the biological innovations that will bolster mental health prevention efforts in children, modern statistics are making it possible to get a better handle on the efficacy and effectiveness of psychosocial interventions. In a seminal study on violence prevention, Sampson, Raudenbush,

* Portions of this article were presented as a workshop at the American Psychiatric Association's 157th Annual Meeting, New York, NY, May 4, 2004.

and Earls (1997) note that in communities with collective efficacy (a measure for social fabric or formal and informal social control) there is less violence, indicating a healthier community. Flay et al. (2004) have also shown the efficacy of psychosocial interventions using modern statistics.

Thus, this new understanding and resultant technology should allow psychiatry to take the lead in constructing a children's mental health and wellness infrastructure that will emphasize early detection and prevention of mental illness (Bell and McKay, 2004). Unfortunately, former Surgeon General Satcher's children's mental health report (U.S. Public Health Service, 2000) notes mental health care is dispersed across multiple systems: schools, primary care providers, the juvenile justice system, child welfare agencies, and substance abuse treatment providers. Thus, the mental health services delivered to children are fragmented. Considering the need for a children's mental health and wellness infrastructure and the current fragmentation of the system, this paper seeks to address how the juvenile justice system will assess and serve the youth under its care.

Although mental health researchers publish little about the incidence and prevalence of mental illness in juvenile detention and correctional facilities (Bell, 2005), there are a handful of studies that focus on the epidemiology of mental illness in juvenile detention centers. The findings from these limited studies are potentially ominous. Cocozza (1992) estimates the rates of mental illness in kids in juvenile detention centers is two to three times higher than in the general population, with about 20% of youth in juvenile detention centers having a serious mental disorder and half of them with co-occurring mental health and substance abuse disorders. The prevalence rates of psychiatric disorders of juvenile offenders have been estimated as: psychoses, 1–6%; affective disorders, 32–78%; anxiety disorders, 6–41%; mental retardation, 7–15%; substance abuse/dependency, 25–95%; learning disorders, 17%; specific developmental disabilities, 53%; attention-deficit hyperactive disorders, 19–46%; and conduct disorder, 50–90% (Abram, Teplin, McClelland, and Dulcan, 2003; National Commission on Correctional Health Care, 2004). In addition, youth suicides in juvenile detention and correctional facilities are occurring four times more often than youth suicide in the general population (Memory, 1989). Yet, 75 percent of the nation's confined juveniles are in facilities that fail to conform to even the most basic suicide prevention guidelines (Bell, 2005). Furthermore, several studies note that a quarter of incarcerated boys and half of the incarcerated girls meet criteria for posttraumatic stress disorder (Burton, Foy, Bwanausi, Johnson, and Moore, 1994).

The following section presents an example of a local-level program which links services of multiple agencies for youth entering the criminal justice system. Independent assessment has found the program successful at maintaining youth in the community.

Mental Health Juvenile Justice (MHJJ) initiative

A large number of youth who come in contact with the juvenile justice system require mental health treatment (Cocozza and Skowyra, 2000), and there is a growing sense of crisis concerning youth involved with the juvenile justice system who are experiencing mental health problems. A number of factors are involved in generating this concern, including: (a) a growing recognition of the mental health needs of youth in general, (b) an increased reliance on the justice center to care for individuals with mental illness, and (c) recent changes in the juvenile justice centers resulting in more youths being transferred to criminal court at younger ages and receiving longer sentences (Cocozza and Skowyra, 2000). Additionally, a series of investigations undertaken by the U.S. Department of Justice into the conditions of confinement in juvenile correctional facilities have repeatedly found a failure on the part of the facilities to adequately address the mental health needs of youth in their care (National Policy Forum on Mental Health and Juvenile Justice, 2003). Mental illness is a serious problem within the juvenile justice system. The fact that many of these disorders are treatable compels us to design a system that identifies at-risk persons and accurately diagnoses disorders and implements corrective action (Bell and Williamson, 2001). For many of these youth, effective treatment that would result in better outcomes, less recidivism, and less offense escalation is not available.

The Mental Health Juvenile Justice (MHJJ) initiative is a collaboration between the Community Mental Health Council Inc. and the Division of Mental Health's Juvenile Forensic Program and it is funded by the Illinois Department of Human Services. The MHJJ initiative is intended to respond to the growing body of research demonstrating that youth in the juvenile justice system suffer from untreated mental health conditions. This program works to respond to the needs of these individuals by providing screening and linkage services to youths in the juvenile justice system who are identified as experiencing a major mental illness. The program targets youth who have been involved with a detention center within the past year and who also exhibit at least one symptom that may indicate a mood or psychotic disorder.

The program provides comprehensive, strength-focused treatment that is culturally sensitive and empirically based. There are several unique aspects of the MHJJ program that contribute to its effectiveness with this population. The child and family are supported with referrals in an effort to maintain the child at home in the community and to prevent the return of the child to a detention center. The clinician works with the family to identify appropriate community services to address mental health treatment, substance abuse treatment, special education, and public health services. This often requires direct interaction with child psychiatrists, child psychologists, parent advocates, and other qualified mental health professionals. The clinician's role is limited to referring a child to appropriate services and serving as a liaison. Services provided often include mental health services, psychological services, educational services, job training, and linkage to recreational activities. The clinician is not involved in legal issues such as a) fitness to participate in legal proceedings or b) insanity evaluations, nor does the clinician function as a therapist. Another strength of this program is the effective utilization of flex funding for services and supports which are tied to the action plan but cannot be afforded by the family. Treatment is limited to six months. However, referrals are designed to provide lasting support and, as such, the program functions to provide long-term treatment planning.

The youth are identified once they enter the juvenile justice system. The juveniles in detention are referred by court personnel to be assessed by a clinician from a community agency. Referrals are made by attorneys, judges, probation staff, and detention center personnel. This allows detention centers to provide access to specialized treatment services while the juvenile is in crisis or in an active phase of his/her problems. This is a time when both the juvenile and his/her parents are the most likely to want to participate in treatment and may provide a good platform from which to initiate the development of a supportive and therapeutic network (Redding, 2000). The juvenile then undergoes an assessment that utilizes several empirically supported assessment tools to address strengths, needs, functioning, and psychiatric illness. The Child and Adolescent Functional Assessment Scale (CAFAS) is a rating scale that assesses the youth's degree of impairment in functioning due to emotional, behavioral, or psychiatric problems (Hodges, 1994). The Child and Adolescent Needs and Strengths (CANS) is an information integration tool designed to support individual case planning and the planning and evaluation of service systems (Lyons et al., 1990). The Childhood Severity of Psychiatric Illness (CSPI) is a tool that is designed to provide a structured assessment of children with possible mental health–service needs along a set of dimensions found to be relevant to clinical decision-making (Lyons, 1998). Referrals for treatment and other services are made, based upon the findings of these and other assessment materials.

Results

The Mental Health Services and Policy Program at Northwestern University Medical School conducted an evaluation of the Mental Health Juvenile Justice initiative after three years of operation. This evaluation concluded that the MHJJ program successfully identified youth who have more mental health problems, engage in riskier behaviors, and have poorer functioning than youth who did not qualify for the program (Lyons, et al., 2003). The results indicate that 27.2% of youth who received MHJJ services in FY03 were rearrested, compared to a 75% rearrest rate for juveniles not receiving treatment. Among MHJJ participants, youth who received more services were less likely to be arrested than other clients. Furthermore, the study concluded that the MHJJ initiative successfully identified youth with serious psychotic and affective disturbances, reduced recidivism, and successfully linked clients to necessary services (Lyons et al., 2003). The MHJJ initiative is an active example of an empirically and community-based approach to addressing the treatment needs of the growing number of youths with mental illness who are entering this country's juvenile justice system. Continued identification of at-risk youth and implementation of community-based, effective approaches to intervention are warranted.

In order to better serve mentally ill youth in the criminal justice system with evidence-based methods, we must have a better understanding of their needs. Research requires resources of time, personnel, and money, all of which are in limited supply. By utilizing data collected during previously established screenings, we can avoid adding to the workload burden but still further the field with research efforts. The next chapter will provide an example of such an effort.

Summary

Clearly, attention is warranted for mentally ill youth in the criminal justice system as public health and social concerns. Multiple government agencies carry mandates to provide services for their communities' youth, but often lack a unifying structure to do so. In times of limited personnel and financial resources, efforts must be made to be efficient without losing effectiveness in providing services. This chapter has highlighted the magnitude of the issue and has illustrated methods of linking services for practical application. Subsequent chapters will describe how to conduct research in order to increase understanding, in an evidence-based manner, with both efforts serving the local community and the field as a whole; and will explore the potential risk of cataloging an information database about juveniles as it relates to sex offenders and their offenses. In an effort to make data available to help society as a whole, one must not forget the impact on the future of that society—the individual children.

Acknowledgments

We acknowledge the Juvenile Justice Issues Corresponding Committee of the American Psychiatric Association for supporting the workshop proposal and the American Psychiatric Association/Shire* Child and Adolescent Psychiatry Fellowship Program Staff for support of the component workshop upon which this article was based in part.

References

Abram, K., Teplin, L., McClelland, G. & Dulcan, M. (2003), Comorbid psychiatric disorders in youth in juvenile detention. *Arch. Gen. Psychiat.*, 60:1097–1108.

Beardslee, W., Gladstone, T., Wright, E. & Cooper, A. (2003), A family-based approach to the prevention of depressive symptoms in children at risk: Evidence of parental and child change. *Pediatrics*, 112:119–131.

Bell, C. (2005), Correctional psychiatry. In *Comprehensive Textbook of Psychiatry*, 8th ed. B. Sadock & V. Sadock. Baltimore: Williams & Wilkins p. 4002–4012.

---

* Program is supported by an unrestricted educational grant from Shire Pharmaceuticals, overseen by the American Psychiatric Association Council on Children, Adolescents, and Their Families, and administered by the Project Director of the Office of Children's Affairs.

Bell, C. & McKay, M. (2004), Constructing a children's mental health infrastructure using community psychiatry principles. *J. Legal Med.*, 25:5–22.

Bell, C. & Williamson, J. (2001), The need for psychiatric infrastructure. *Paradigm Magazine*, 6:14–15, 19.

Bhana, A., Petersen, I., Mason, A., Mahintsho, Z., Bell, C., & McKay, M. (2004), Children and youth at risk: Adaptation and pilot study of the CHAMP (Amaqhawe) programme in South Africa. *African J. AIDS Research (AJAR)*, 3:33–41.

Burton, D., Foy, D., Bwanausi, C., Johnson, J., & Moore, L. (1994). The relationship between traumatic exposure, family dysfunction, and post-traumatic stress symptoms in male juvenile offenders. *J. Traumatic Stress*, 7:83–92.

Charney, D. (2004), Psychobiological mechanisms of resilience and vulnerability: Implications for successful adaptation to extreme stress. *Am. J. Psychiat.*, 161: 195–216.

Cocozza, J., ed. (1992), *Responding to the Mental Health Needs of Youth in the Juvenile Justice System.* Seattle, WA: The National Coalition for the Mentally Ill in the Criminal Justice System.

Cocozza, J. & Skowyra, K. (2000), Youth with mental health disorders: Issues and emerging responses. *Juvenile Justice*, 7:3–13.

Flay, B., Graumlich, S., Segawa, E., Burns, J., Amuwo, S., Bell, C., Campbell, R., Cowell, J., Cooksey, J., Dancy, B., Hedeker, D., Jagers, R., Levy, S., Paikoff, R., Punwani, I., & Weisberg, R. (2004), The ABAN AYA Youth Project: Effects of comprehensive prevention programs on high risk behaviors among inner city African American youth: A randomized trial. *Arch. Peds. Adolesc. Med.*, 158:377–384.

Hodges, K. (1994), *Child and Adolescent Functional Assessment Scale,* revised ed. Ypsilanti, MI: Eastern Michigan University Department of Psychology. (Originally published in 1990)

Lyons, J. (1998), *The Severity of Psychiatric Illness Scale—Child and Adolescent Version.* San Antonio, TX: Psychological Corp.

Lyons, J., Griffin, E., Fazio, M., & Lyons, M. B. (1999), *The Child and Adolescent Needs and Strengths: An Information Integration Tool for Children With Mental Health Challenges and Their Families.* Chicago: Northwestern University Institute for Health Services Research and Policy Studies.

Lyons, J., Griffin, G., Quintenz, S., Jenuwine, M., & Shasha, M. (2003), Clinical and forensic outcomes from the Illinois mental health juvenile justice initiative. *Psychiatr. Serv.*, 54:1629–34.

McFarlane, W. (2001), Family-based treatment in prodromal and first-episode psychosis. In *Early Intervention in Psychotic Disorders*, ed. T. Miller. Amsterdam, Netherlands: Kluwer Academic Publishers, pp. 197–230.

Memory, J. (1989), Juvenile suicides in secure detention facilities: Correction of published rates, *Death Studies*, 13:455–463.

National Commission on Correctional Health Care (2004), *The Health Status of Soon-To-Be-Released Inmates.* Chicago: National Commission on Correctional Health Care.

National Policy Forum on Mental Health and Juvenile Justice. (2003), *Moving Toward an Integrated Policy for Youth.* Delmar, NY: National Center for Mental Health and Juvenile Justice.

Redding, R. E. (2000), Barriers to meeting the mental health needs of offenders in the juvenile justice system. *Juvenile Justice Fact Sheet.* Charlottesville, VA: University of Virginia Institute of Law, Psychiatry, & Public Policy.

Sampson, R., Raudenbush, R., & Earls, F. (1997), Neighborhoods and violent crime: A multilevel study of collective efficacy. *Science*, 277:918–924.

U.S. Public Health Service (USPHA) (2000), *Report of the Surgeon General's Conference on Children's Mental Health: A National Action Agenda*. Washington, DC: Department of Health and Human Services.

5 The mandatory registration of juvenile sex offenders and commitment of juveniles as sexually violent predators

Controversies and recommendations*

Richard L. Frierson, R. Gregg Dwyer, Carl C. Bell, and Johnny L. Williamson

Abstract

This chapter explores the potential risks of cataloging a database of information about juveniles as it relates to sex offenders and their offenses.

The information gathered during a juvenile offender's incarceration can be used to identify mental illness, to individualize mental health treatment, to link the juvenile with a variety of treatment resources, and to plan for future mental health treatment after the juvenile offender leaves a correctional facility. The immediate goal of each of these data utilization venues is the provision of appropriate and successful mental health treatment. The ultimate goal of these venues is to prevent future recidivism. Although juvenile offenders are presumed to benefit from assessment and treatment, the protection of society from further harmful acts is inherent in both of these goals. The evaluation of juvenile sex offenders is particularly fraught with implications for society as well as for the juvenile's future life.

Significant recidivism is common in adult sex offenders (Prentky, 1997) and has also been encountered among the juvenile sex offender population (Worling, 2000). Because of these high recidivism rates, numerous jurisdictions and the federal government have enacted laws aimed at preventing recidivism and protecting the public at large from future victimization once sex offenders are released from custody. Information gathered from juvenile sex offenders, including the presence of sexual disorders (i.e., paraphilia), conduct disorder, other mental illness, or prior sexual assaults not known to the criminal justice system, can be used to trigger a juvenile's referral to a sex-offender registry or to a civil commitment process commonly known as sexually violent offender (SVO) or sexually violent predator (SVP) commitment. Frequently, these laws have been the subject of controversy, especially when applied to juvenile offenders, and have been challenged in both state and federal courts. This chapter will review two types of these laws: laws requiring sex offender registration with or without community notification,

---

* Portions of this article were presented as a workshop at the American Psychiatric Association's 157th Annual Meeting, New York, NY, May 4, 2004.

and laws committing sex offenders to sex offender treatment at the time they are released from incarceration. Problems associated with the application of these laws to juveniles will also be discussed.

Sex offender registration

The governmental goals of sex offender registration are threefold: to deter previous offenders from committing future crimes by having offenders monitored by police, to provide law enforcement with an additional investigative tool to identify potential suspects in new sexual assault cases, and to increase public awareness of and public self-protection from crimes against children.

The history of sexual offender registration laws begins at the state level. These initial sex offender registration laws were frequently enacted following a high-profile case of childhood sexual assault. In 1989, 11-year-old Jacob Wetterling was abducted by a masked man and never found. His parents successfully lobbied all 50 states to establish sex offender registries. These laws became known as the Wetterling Act (Jacob Wetterling Crimes Against Children and Sex Offender Registration Act, 1994). The Federal Violent Crime Control and Law Enforcement Act of 1994 incorporated the Wetterling Act and required the establishment of sex offender registries in all 50 states. It also required offenders to register their address annually for 10 years (Federal Violent Crime Act, 1994). Furthermore, this law allowed for but did not require information about a registrant's prior offenses to be released to the public. In 1994, 7-year-old Megan Nichole Kanka was lured with a puppy to a neighbor's home and was subsequently brutally raped and murdered by a twice-convicted sex offender who had previously assaulted a 5-year-old and a 7-year-old child. In response to this high profile crime, a federal law known as Megan's Law was passed which amended the Wetterling Act to require that all 50 states "shall release relevant information as necessary to protect the public" (Megan's Law, 1996). However, this law did not mandate active community notification (door-to-door notification, direct mailings, fax and computer transmissions, media notices, etc.), and the majority of states only actively notify on a case-by-case basis. Finally, in 1996 Congress passed the Pam Lyncher Act, an amendment to the Wetterling Act that requires offenders who have been convicted of an aggravated sex offense or multiple registerable offenses to be subject to lifetime registration. Furthermore, the Lyncher amendment required the U.S. Attorney General to establish a database at the Federal Bureau of Investigation (FBI) to track the whereabouts and movements of certain convicted sex offenders (*Pam Lyncher Act, 1996*).

There have been numerous constitutional challenges to sex offender registration. Most of these cases have challenged these laws as a violation of the U.S. Constitution's ex post facto clause. The U.S. Supreme Court has held that due process does not require a showing of dangerousness before an offender is placed on a registry because placement on a registry does not violate a liberty interest, including damage to the registrant's reputation (Connecticut Dept. of Public

Safety v. Doe, 2003). In a later case, the Court held that "our system does not treat dissemination of truthful information in furtherance of a legitimate governmental objective as punishment" (Smith v. Doe, 2003).

Currently, 38 states include the registration of juvenile sex offenders in their sex offender registries without restrictions. Alaska, Florida, and Maine will register juveniles only if they were tried as an adult. Indiana registers juveniles age 14 and older. South Dakota registers juveniles age 15 and older. New Hampshire, New Mexico, Utah, and Wyoming only register individuals age 18 and older and Alabama only registers individuals 20 years and older. Finally, Mississippi only registers juveniles with two sexual offense convictions (Klaass Kids Foundation, 2004).

Most states allow public access to sex offender registries via the Internet. These registries allow anyone with a computer to locate registered sex offenders who live in their neighborhood or area. Most of these registries also allow searches by name. Fifteen states have elected not to provide access to registries via the Internet: California, Colorado, Hawaii, Idaho, Maine, Massachusetts, Missouri, Nevada, New Hampshire, North Dakota, Oklahoma, Pennsylvania, Rhode Island, South Dakota, and Washington (Federal Bureau of Investigation).

Sexually violent predator statutes

In 1990, Washington became the first state to enact a modern Sexually Violent Predator Act. Since that time, at least 18 states (Arizona, California, Florida, Illinois, Iowa, Kansas, Massachusetts, Minnesota, Missouri, New Jersey, North Dakota, Pennsylvania, South Carolina, Texas, Vermont, Virginia, Washington, and Wisconsin) have enacted similar statutes—frequently referred to as sexual predator laws—which provide for involuntary commitment of violent sex offenders after they have completed their prison sentences (Tucker & Brakel, 2003). This commitment occurs indefinitely and can also be applied to those individuals found incompetent to stand trial or legally insane at the time of their offense. Like the sex offender registry laws, these commitment laws have also been constitutionally challenged. However, courts have declared that these acts are not criminal in nature and aim to provide treatment for the offender; therefore there is no double jeopardy or violation of the ex post facto clause (Kansas v. Hendricks, 1997). The U.S. Supreme Court has also held that the State does not have to show that the offender had a complete lack of ability to control behavior, but only significant difficulty: "The line between an irresistible impulse and an impulse not resisted is probably no sharper than that between twilight and dusk" (Kansas v. Crane, 2002). The majority of these statutes allow for the commitment of juvenile offenders as sexually violent predators.

The inclusion of juveniles

The application of these laws to juvenile sex offenders is controversial. Should data obtained from a juvenile offender be used to refer the juvenile to a sex offender registry or a sexually violent predator commitment process? Proponents argue that the goal of protecting potential future victims is paramount and these laws act as deterrents to future offending and provide an investigative tool to law enforcement agencies (Center for Sex Offender Management, 1999. Furthermore, these laws allow ongoing monitoring by authorities and allow for employment security checks for day cares, schools, and child-oriented businesses.

There are also criticisms of the application of these laws to juveniles. The referral of a juvenile to a registry can create significant stigma as the juvenile becomes labeled. Consequently after having successfully completed sex offender treatment, the juvenile may have significant difficulty reintegrating into an education system if the offender's peers become aware of his or her appearance on a registry. Recently, an author of this chapter consulted on a 12-year-old girl with significantly delayed social skills who was convicted of Lewd Act on a Minor after she was found playing with several 6-year-old children in her neighborhood and they had all removed their clothing. She could not return to her school of origin after her picture was picked up from her state's internet sex offender registry and was posted around the school by her peers. Because one of the goals of most sex offender treatment programs is the development of appropriate peer relationships, the stigma created by inclusion in a registry may actually hinder this important treatment goal. Secondly, many assessment techniques used with adult offenders—penile plethysmography, for example—have not been validated or standardized on juvenile offenders. Thus there is a risk of inappropriate assignment of a diagnosis of a sexual disorder. Finally, juvenile sex offenders represent a heterogeneous group. Sexually abused younger children frequently manifest sexually aggressive behaviors, particularly towards other children. Many young adolescents may engage in sexual experimentation with younger peers, but do not develop recurrent pedophilic fantasies.

Potential approaches to prevent data misuse

The use of data gathered from juvenile sex offenders during incarceration is currently used indiscriminately in the creation of sex offender registries and in the referral of juveniles to sexually violent predator commitment. However, these offenders represent a very heterogeneous group. One typology of juvenile sex offenders has suggested four subtypes: a) an offender with a true paraphilia, b) an antisocial youth whose sex offending is merely one facet of the exploitation of others, c) a juvenile compromised by a psychiatric or neurobiological disorder who has poor impulse control as a result of his/her condition, and d) a youth with impaired social and interpersonal skills who turns to younger children for sexual gratification (Shaw, 2002).

Indiscriminate referrals of juvenile sex offenders may result in the registration or commitment of some offenders who do not represent a significant threat of future recidivism. Unnecessary civil commitments can waste financial and treatment resources. More selective approaches should be considered. One potential approach would involve requiring age limits (over 15 years, for example) before a juvenile is registered or committed. An alternative might require that there be multiple offenses. Another approach would be to require a juvenile offender be convicted in adult court before being referred for registration or commitment. Finally, the evaluation of juveniles on a case by case basis with a formal risk assessment and review at a formal hearing may help prevent the unnecessary registration or commitment of nonviolent juveniles. These risk assessments should be conducted using scientific evidence regarding the risk factors for reoffending. Such an approach should lead to consideration of case-specific variables that are ignored in many cases. For example, it may be inappropriate to register or commit a 17-year-old juvenile sex offender who has Klinefelter's disorder and whose single sex offense occurred against a family member while he was receiving testosterone replacement therapy. The aforementioned 12-year-old girl might also pose little risk for reoffending and could be viewed as inappropriate for placement on a registry or commitment as a sexually violent predator. However, a 14-year-old male, with two separate sex offenses against small children and who reports deviant sexual interests and has abnormal arousal patterns on penile plethysmography (PPG) and other measures of deviant sexual interest that have been standardized in a juvenile population sample, might be appropriate for referral to a registry or for treatment of a developing paraphilia. As stated previously in this chapter, caution is warranted in the interpretation of PPGs and other measures of deviant sexual interest as many of the PPG stimulus sets and other tests of deviant interest have not been normalized for use on adolescents. This underscores a potential barrier to individualized risk assessments: the lack of professionals trained in the evaluation of juvenile sex offenders. Unfortunately, organized medical education in child and adolescent psychiatry has ignored this problem. While emphasis is placed on the evaluation and treatment of children who are victims of sexual abuse, much less attention is paid to juvenile perpetrators of sexual abuse. Child and adolescent residency program requirements fail to mention the assessment or treatment of juvenile sex offenders (Accreditation Council for Graduate Medical Education, 2005). Because juvenile sex offenders are a heterogeneous population, specialized skill and training is needed for competent assessment.

As we have described in the previous chapter, efforts are underway to further our understanding of juvenile sex offenders. In that chapter, Williamson and colleagues (in press) report the results of research in progress from a study that compares juvenile sex offenders to other juvenile offenders in a detention setting by using data originally collected as part of the study agency's initial mental health screening. Although findings are preliminary, statistically significant differences were discovered.

The screening instrument utilized was not designed, nor were there any indications it was being used in the study setting, for discriminating juveniles who sexually offended from those who did not. Rather the goal of the reported research was to seek new sources of mental health data for use in developing a practical typology of adolescent sexual offenders, in order to make distinctions among offenders in the context of treatment planning and prevention programs. Although the research goal is clearly focused on advancing the field's understanding of a specific segment of the juvenile justice population, caution must be exercised so that data collected for mental health purposes is not used in a manner detrimental to the youth being studied.

Unfortunately, the causes and course of sexual offending (including recidivism) and the paraphilias have been largely limited to adults (Saleh, 2004). Further research on juvenile sex offenders is clearly needed. In an effort to make data available to help society as a whole, one must not forget the impact on the future of that society—the individual children.

References

Pam Lyncher Sexual Offender Tracking and Identification Act 42 U.S.C. 14072 (1996).

Accreditation Council for Graduate Medical Education (ACGME). *Program requirements for residency education in child and adolescent psychiatry.* Available at http:// www.acgme.org/acWebsite/downloads/RRC_progReq/405pr1104.pdf. Accessed September 12, 2005.

Center for Sex Offender Management, United States Department of Justice. Sex offender registration: Policy overview and comprehensive practices, 1999. Retrieved September 10, 2005 at http://www.csom.org/pubs/sexreg.pdf.

Connecticut Department of Public Safety v. Doe, 123 S. Ct. 1160 (2003).

Federal Bureau of Investigation. Investigative programs crimes against children. Retrieved January 21, 2005 from http://www.fbi.gov/hq/cid/cac/states.htm.

Federal Violent Crime and Law Enforcement Act, 42 U.S.C. 13701 (1994).

Jacob Wetterling Crimes Against Children and Sex Offender Registration Act, 42 U.S.C. 14071 §170101 (1994).

Kansas v. Crane, 534 U.S. 407 (2002).

Kansas v. Hendricks, 521 U.S. 346 (1997).

KlaasKids Foundation, (2004). Megan's Law by state. Retrieved January 19, 2005 at http:// www.klaaskids.org/pg-legmeg.htm.

Megan's Law, 42 U.S.C. 13701, Pub. L. 104–145, Section 1, May 17, 1996, 110 Stat. 1345.

Prentky, R., Lee, A., Knight, R. & Cerce, D. (1997), Recidivism rates among child molesters and rapists: A methodological analysis. *Law and Human Behavior,* 21:635–659.

Saleh, F. & Vincent, G. (2004), Juveniles who commit sex crimes. *Adolescent Psychiatry,* 28:183–207.

Shaw, J. (2002), Sexually aggressive youth. In *Principles and practice of child and adolescent forensic psychiatry,* ed. D. Schetky and E. Benedek. Washington DC: American Psychiatric Publishing, Inc., pp. 279–287.

Smith v. Doe, 123 S. Ct. 1140 (2003).

Tucker, D. & Brakel, S. (2003), Sexually violent predator laws, In *Principles and Practice of Forensic Psychiatry,* 2nd ed., ed. R. Rosner. London, England: Arnold Publishers, pp. 717–723.

Williamson, J. L., Bell, C. C., Dwyer, R. G. & Frierson, R. L. (in press), Toward a better juvenile justice system. In: *Adolescent Psychiatry,* ed. L. T. Flaherty. Mahwah, NJ: The Analytic Press.

Worling, J. & Curwen T. (2000), Adolescent sexual offender recidivism: Success of specialized treatment and implications for risk prediction. *Child Abuse Negl.*, 24:965–982.

6 Use of assessment data for research in juvenile justice*
An exploratory study of sex offenders

R. Gregg Dwyer, Carl C. Bell, Richard L. Frierson, and Johnny L. Williamson

Note: The South Carolina Department of Juvenile Justice (SCDJJ) data was provided with the agreement that subjects' identities would be concealed. Data was not released by the SCDJJ until de-identified. The SCDJJ has no responsibility for the statistical analysis or conclusions derived therefrom and presented in this paper.

Abstract

An existing psychiatric assessment system within the South Carolina Department of Juvenile Justice (SCDJJ) was utilized as a data source for conducting a study to identify differences between detained juvenile sex offenders and non-sex offenders across mental health parameters, to identify the need for mental health treatment among detained juvenile sex offenders, and to reveal areas of value for future research. The preliminary results of a study that compared juvenile sex offenders to other juvenile offenders are presented to illustrate the use of screening and assessment data for alternative uses, namely furthering the field's understanding of a segment of the juvenile population.

Assessment and screening

The April, 2002, Consensus Conference on Juvenile Justice Mental Health Assessments (Wasserman et al., 2003) proposed several recommendations regarding assessment. These included (a) mental health screening within twenty-four hours of arrival at a facility, (b) mental health screening and assessment as soon as possible after arrival to identify mental health service needs, (c) assessment with multiple sources of information and measurement of a range of concerns, (d) screening and assessment upon discharge from a facility and return to the community, (e) screening and assessment on a regular basis, and (f) screening and assessments conducted by credentialed mental health staff or by persons directly

---

* Portions of this article were presented as a workshop at the American Psychiatric Association's 157th Annual Meeting, New York, NY, May 4, 2004.

supervised by credentialed staff trained in screening and assessment. Screening is defined as "the identification of unrecognized problems in apparently well persons via procedures that can be applied rapidly and inexpensively" (pg 753).

The South Carolina Department of Juvenile Justice (SCDJJ) is the agency responsible for "rehabilitation and custodial care to juveniles" on probation, incarcerated, or on parole for a criminal or status offense (SCDJJ, 2004). The agency's policies mandate that an initial assessment be conducted to screen for safety of the juveniles and staff, to identify serious mental illness and/or mental retardation, and to obtain data for treatment planning (W. Haxton, personal communication, April 23, 2004).* Within one hour of arrival, juveniles are asked brief general medical and mental health questions by a nonclinician. An on-call clinician is available as needed. Within forty-eight hours, the Massachusetts Youth Screening Instrument™, Version 2 (MAYSI™–2) is administered. The juvenile's available medical and educational records are reviewed as well as the juvenile's current psychiatric diagnosis and medications.

The MAYSI™–2, a fifty-two yes/no-question self-report instrument was designed to screen twelve-to seventeen-year-olds for mental health needs at the entry level and transition stages in a juvenile justice system (Grisso and Barnum, 2003). The MAYSI™–2 is composed of seven scales that assess risks in the following areas: reaction to no access to alcohol and/or drugs; angry reactions, fights, and aggression; depression and anxiety disorders; psychological distress with somatic complaints; suicide attempts or gestures; thought disorder; and exposure to trauma (Grisso and Barnum, 2003). The scale scores are designed to raise a red flag, but cutoff scores are decided at each agency's discretion (Grisso and Barnum, 2003). The MAYSI™–2 test-retest correlations have been reported as stable, over a brief period of time, compared to other screening instruments designed for use with youths. Prior studies indicate that there is general construct validity for the scales (Grisso and Barnum, 2003). Gender (Grisso and Barnum, 2003; Stewart and Trupin, 2003) and ethnic differences have been found in MAYSI™–2 results (Stewart and Trupin, 2003; Grisso, Barnum, Fletcher, Cauffman, and Peuschold, 2001) with the ethnic differences being viewed as possible artifact, actual mental health differences, or differences in referrals based on bias.

Methods

A retrospective design was used to compare juvenile sex offenders (SO subjects) to non-sex offenders (non-SO subjects) in the residential levels of the SCDJJ. Equivalent Institutional Review Board (IRB) approval was provided by the SCDJJ Research and Statistics Department that was performing the agency's IRB function at the time this research proposal was submitted. Existing MAYSI™–2 raw data was accessed for all admissions from October 1999 to June 2003, per-

---

* William Haxton, Director of Clinical and Professional Services, South Carolina Department of Juvenile Justice.

sonal identifying data was removed, and female non-sex offenders were deleted from the data set because the SCDJJ Sex Offender Treatment Program (SOTP) program did not include females. Obtained frequencies included age, ethnicity, SCDJJ facility, MAYSI™–2 raw scores, and MAYSI™–2 scale scores for the 2215 non-SO subjects and 45 SO subjects after deletions. Cross tabulations, Pearson Chi-Square, Likelihood Ratio, Fischer's Exact Test, ANOVA, logistic regression, multiple regression, and ordinal LOGIT models were employed. Analysis included assessment of relationships between ethnicity, facility, responses to individual MAYSI™–2 questions, MAYSI™–2 raw scores, and MAYSI™–2 scale scores and status as being a SO or not being a SO; relationships between raw scores for each MAYSI™–2 scale and non-SO and SO status; and relationships between the MAYSI™–2 scale scores and age and ethnicity.

Results

Assessment data from the MAYSI™–2 provided information for furthering understanding and for future research relative to sex offending and non-sex offending juveniles. Although few, the differences revealed raise some interesting questions about juvenile sex offenders. Given the exploratory nature of this study and the focus of this article on data use in a service setting, only the highlights and preliminary suggestions from the research are provided at this time as an example of alternative uses for practice-based data.

The mean age for the non-SO juveniles was 15.2 years old (std dev 1.272) and for the SO subjects was 14.7 years old (std dev 1.255). Non-SO youths were 1.3 times more likely to be older than SO participants ($p = 0.018$). When controlled for ethnicity, this difference was maintained ($p = 0.018$, 95% CI = 0.595, 0.953). This age distribution was consistent with that reported by previous research. The lower mean age for the sex offenders raises the question of whether or not sex offenders are likely to be held in residential settings at a younger age than juveniles who commit other types of offenses.

There were no statistical differences between the SO and non-SO juveniles when considered alone on the basis of ethnicity, SCDJJ system level (detention, evaluation, and orientation), or the seven MAYSI™–2 scales, but significant and nearly significant differences were found among individual question responses between SO and non-SO youths. A summary of those findings follows. Approaching statistical significance was the finding that SOs were 1.8 times more likely than non-SOs to indicate that they had easily lost their temper or had a short fuse ($p = 0.057$, $X^2 = 3.636$, df = 1). When controlling for age and ethnicity, SO were 1.9 times more likely to indicate these findings ($p = 0.039$, 95% CI = 1.032, 3.571).

SOs indicated they had been able to make other people do things, just by thinking about it, 2.3 times more than non-SOs ($p = 0.044$, $X^2 = 4.067$, df = 1), but when controlling for age and ethnicity, this significance was lost. Although this item was from the Thought Disturbance Scale and referred to psychotic symptoms, it may have been answered positively because of a misinterpretation of the item as referring to persuasion or coercion of a victim rather than a psychotic symptom.

SOs were 2.3 times more likely to report that they had given up hope for life ($p = 0.022$, $X^2 = 5.244$, df = 1), and when controlled for age and ethnicity SOs were 2.4 times more likely to indicate this ($p = 0.032$, 95% CI = 1.076, 5.310). This item is from the Depressed-Anxious and Suicide Ideation s.cales. The SO juveniles' positive responses could be secondary to the indeterminate sentences that a juvenile sex offender receives with a likely lengthy treatment stay. Also, being labeled a sex offender, possibly for life, with impact on job seeking and interpersonal relationships may contribute to their answers as well. Finally, there may be a higher rate of depressive and/or anxious symptoms and disorders among residentially treated juvenile sex offenders than juveniles with other offenses.

Approaching statistical significance was the finding that SOs were 2.4 times more likely to respond "yes" to being asked if they had ever been raped or in danger of being raped ($p = 0.061$, $X^2 = 3.498$, df = 1), but this significance disappeared when age and ethnicity were controlled. Although designed to be a *female* scale item, addressing sexual victimization or fear of victimization, this finding is not surprising. Shaw et al. (1993) reported that as many as 65% of juvenile sex offenders reported their own histories of sexual victimization. However, Rich (2003) noted that being a victim of sexual abuse does not usually lead to future offending, nor is it common.

Discussion

The main limitation of the study is that it included the use of a relatively small number of male-only detained sex offenders at a single site. Therefore, the lack of differences with some variables could be an accurate representation or a function of the relatively small sample of SO subjects (n = 45). An additional limitation is that the MAYSI™–2 is a self-report instrument allowing for potential reporting bias and data were missing for some subjects (age, ethnicity, and MAYSI™–2 responses), thus limiting the available sample size further. Despite these limitations, the following suggestions are proposed.

In keeping with the September, 2000, Surgeon General's Conference on Children's Mental Health, we should continue to address mental health needs assessment for detained juvenile offenders and work to prevent entry into the justice system through services at the level of "primary care, schools, welfare," and the "larger mental health system" (U. S. Public Health Service, 2000, p. 524). At the community level, by utilizing components of the "rebuilding the village" approach to youth violence (Bell, Flay, and Paikoff, 2002), we should teach social skills; use a multidisciplinary intervention as soon as possible to treat the trauma of sexual victimization; and, when addressing risk management, include protective measures regarding sexual behaviors. Another goal includes heightening awareness of the need among primary care providers to screen for sexual offending behaviors.

Although not specifically designed for use in treatment planning, responses to several questions include areas for treatment focus. Given that SOs were approximately twice as likely to indicate having a quick temper, anger management strategies should be a part of their treatment plan. The SOs were approximately 2.5 times more likely to indicate a loss of hope for their lives. Further assessment and possible treatment with psychotherapy and/or medication of depressive pathology is certainly warranted. Given the potential long-term nature of the stigma associated with their offenses and the average length of their confinement, it seems reasonable to include periodic assessment for depressive symptoms.

As a public health issue, sexual offending warrants the attention of mental health and general medical professionals to help devise methods for primary and secondary prevention and public and professional education. This research effort provides another opportunity to add to our understanding of these mental and physical health care issues and provides both practical prevention suggestions and future research topics. Clearly this use of data, collected about youth, would likely be labeled by most as beneficial and positive. Other uses are more controversial and deserve closer scrutiny by the field. The previous chapter identified an area of concern where the line between benefit and risk is not clearly drawn.

Summary

Clearly, attention is warranted for mentally ill youth in the criminal justice system as public health and social concerns. Multiple government agencies carry mandates to provide services for their communities' youth, but often lack a unifying structure to do so. In times of limited personnel and financial resources, efforts must be made to be efficient without losing effectiveness in providing services. This paper has highlighted the magnitude of the issue and has illustrated methods to a) link services for practical application and b) to conduct research to further understanding in an evidence-based manner, with both efforts serving the local community and the field as a whole.

Acknowledgments

We acknowledge the Juvenile Justice Issues Corresponding Committee of the American Psychiatric Association for supporting the workshop proposal; and the American Psychiatric Association/Shire* Child and Adolescent Psychiatry Fellowship Program Staff for support to the component workshop upon which this article was based in part. This program is supported by an unrestricted educational grant from Shire Pharmaceuticals, overseen by the American Psychiatric Association Council on Children, Adolescents, and Their Families, and administered by the Project Director of the Office of Children's Affairs. Additionally, Dr. Dwyer acknowledges Dr. William Haxton of the South Carolina Department of Juvenile Justice (SCDJJ) for his assistance in obtaining access to SCDJJ data; and Dr. Roumen Vesselinov of the Department of Statistics, University of South Carolina, for his guidance with designing the statistical analysis and assistance with interpreting the results.

References

Bell, C., Flay, B. & Paikoff, R. (2002), Strategies for health behavioral change. In *The Health Behavioral Change Imperative: Theory, Education, and Practice in Diverse Populations*, ed. J. Chunn. New York: Kluwer Academic/Plenum Publishers, pp. 17–39.

Grisso, T. & Barnum, R. (2003), *Massachusetts Youth Screening Instrument™–Version 2: User's Manual and Technical Report*. Sarasota, FL: Professional Resources Press.

Grisso, T., Barnum, R., Fletcher, K., Cauffman, E. & Peuschold, D. (2001), Massachusetts Youth Screening Instrument for mental health needs of juvenile justice youths. *J. Am. Acad. Child. Adolesc. Psychiat.*, 40:541–548.

Rich, P. (2003), *Understanding, Assessing, and Rehabilitating Juvenile Sexual Offenders*. Hoboken, NJ: John Wiley & Sons, Inc.

Shaw, J., Campo-Bowen, A., Applegate, B., Perez, D., Antoine, L., Hart, E., Lahley, B., Testa, R. & Devaney, A. (1993), Young boys who commit serious sexual offenses: Demographics, psychometrics, and phenomenology. *Bull. Am. Acad. Psychiat. Law*, 21:399–408.

South Carolina Department of Juvenile Justice (SCDJJ), *Agency Overview*. Accessed 03/30/04 from http://www.state.sc.us/djj/pdfs/agency-overview.pdf.

Stewart, D. & Trupin, E. (2003), Clinical utility and policy implications of a statewide mental health screening process for juvenile offenders. *Psychiatric Services*, 54:377–382.

U.S. Public Health Service (2000), *Report of the Surgeon General's Conference on Children's Mental Health: A National Action Agenda*. Washington, DC: Department of Health and Human Services.

Wasserman, G., Jensen, P., Ko, S., Cocozza, J., Trupin, E., Angold, A., Cauffman, E. & Grisso, T. (2003), Mental health assessments in juvenile justice: Report on the consensus conference. *J. Am. Acad. Child Adolesc. Psychiat.*, 42:752–761.

7 Residential treatment for gifted and self-destructive adolescents
The John Dewey Academy

Thomas Edward Bratter, Lisa Sinsheimer, Danielle Sara Kaufman, and Jonathan Steven Alter

Abstract

This chapter describes the John Dewey Academy (JDA), its students, and its educational and therapeutic philosophy. It offers a rationale for the efficacy of caring confrontation and the utilization of positive peer pressure within a therapeutic community setting. Psychotropic medications are not used. Outcomes are strongly positive in a population of bright adolescents who are resistant to traditional treatment. We contend that these treatment approaches make the John Dewey Academy unique.

> Here's to the crazy ones.
> The misfits.
> The rebels.
> The troublemakers.
> The round pegs in the square holes.
> The ones who see things differently.
> They're not fond of rules.
> And they have no respect for the status quo.
> You can praise them, disagree with them, quote them,
> disbelieve them, glorify them or vilify them.
> About the only thing you can't do is ignore them.
> Because they change things.
> They invent. They imagine. They heal.
> They explore. They create. They inspire.
> They push the human race forward.
> Maybe they have to be crazy.
> How else can you stare at an empty canvas and see a work of art?
> Or sit in silence and hear a song that's never been written?
> Or gaze at a red planet and see a laboratory on wheels?
> Because the people who are crazy enough to think they
>   can change the world, are the ones who do.
>
> **Anonymous poem by a student**

The school and its students

Founded in 1985, the John Dewey Academy (JDA) is a therapeutic boarding school based on the concept of caring confrontation and self-help positive peer pressure within a therapeutic community setting (Bratter, Bratter, Maxym, and Steiner, 1998). JDA's primary identification is a college preparatory residential high school for grades 10–12. It provides intensive education and treatment for approximately 30 self-destructive adolescents who have failed to respond to other treatment approaches.

Admission criteria and student characteristics

Admission is determined on the basis of in-person interviews after a telephone interview with parents. There are four criteria that determine acceptability: (1) possessing the potential to succeed; (2) having the energy to succeed; (3) agreeing to become a contributing member of the community; and (4) wanting to attend college. We exclude prior educational performance, standardized test scores, and psychological reports. Approximately, seventy-five percent of those whom we interview are admitted.

We do not put much stock in prior testing and school reports, as these are often distorted by lack of motivation and/or substance abuse, and may not assess academic potential. At base, our program is a meritocracy. Students arrive, however, looking anything but meritorious.

The John Dewey Academy is not appropriate for all adolescents. Those who are organically damaged, have *true* metabolic disorders, possess less than average intelligence, and/or are psychotic are not considered viable candidates.

Referral sources

Interestingly, less than ten percent of our referrals come from mental health specialists. We believe this stems from our uncompromising opposition toward the use of psychotropic medications and diagnostic labels. Significantly, twenty percent of Dewey graduates have at least one parent who works as a psychotherapist. Most families learn about the John Dewey Academy from the Internet or from independent educational consultants they have hired to help when other treatment approaches have not worked. Now that the school is over twenty years old, we have developed a strong word-of-mouth referral base from alumni and alumni parents.

Student characteristics

Many students arrive at JDA with educational deficiencies, functioning one or more grades below chronological age. More than 90% have inconsistent and mediocre academic records, and most have inferior standardized test scores. Students who enter have stolen, cheated, lied, betrayed, manipulated those around them, and have rejected traditional psychotherapeutic and pedological approaches. These youngsters have been branded by family, friends, therapists, and teachers as untreatable, uneducable, unreliable, unmanageable, unruly, uncivilized, untrust-worthy, unlovable, unworthy, unwanted, undisciplined, unfaithful, unpredictable, unhappy, unlawful, unstable, and unsuccessful.

Prior to their admission, 33% of the students have been hospitalized or attended drug and alcohol treatment programs for one month, 75% have been treated by mental health specialists, and 50% arrive medicated with potent psychotropics. They bear a myriad of DSM-IV diagnoses given by inpatient programs and com-munity-based psychotherapists. Some of the more common diagnoses include: bipolar affective disorder, major depressive disorder, oppositional defiant disor-der, attention deficit hyperactivity disorder, and various substance use disorders. In summary, these children have been labeled with multiple and very severe dis-orders, and have been medicated accordingly. This is part of the insidious trend in psychiatry and education that involves labeling disruptive and disobedient stu-dents with attention-deficit disorders or conduct disorders, or even bipolar disor-ders (Harris, 2005).

By the time they arrive at Dewey, these youngsters are often psychological cripples, hiding behind their diagnostic shields and excuses. Furthermore, these labels can haunt the possessor in adulthood when applying for a driver's license, life insurance, licensure as a professional, and so on.

We believe there are three reasons for the plethora of diagnoses. First, bright and gifted adolescents are irritating so the therapist may give a punitive diagnosis. Second, insurance companies encourage excessive diagnoses to justify payment. Third, in professional journals, certain diagnoses become trends. In contrast to the above excessive diagnoses, our students do not come with the diagnoses they actually meet criteria for. Most of all our students actually *have* nicotine depen-dency and identity problems but none has ever been given either of these diag-noses. Neither has the most benign and inclusive diagnosis, adjustment disorder, been used.

Who these kids really are

These teenagers are unconvinced. They feel that life has nothing worthwhile to offer—"a fundamental psychic problem in circumstances of late modernity" (Giddens, 1991, p. 9). They are motivated by intense emotions they can neither understand nor identify. They create crises and chaos to escape feelings of depres-sion. Some medicate themselves for the temporary relief of painful feelings. Oth-ers are promiscuous to neutralize loneliness. Their symptoms are legion, and are designed to help with the avoidance of painful reality. They include: eating disordered behavior; suicidality and suicidal thinking; self-destructive behav-iors such as cutting, gambling, addiction to the Internet, or to other electronic entertainment; or stealing money or consumer goods. Creating constant crises with self-destructive acts, they need a structured, safe, and supportive residential environment to help them control and curtail their behavior. They are similar to the adolescents with educational deficiencies in secure units that Rose (2004) describes as "likely to be disaffected with or have disengaged from education… and…they may have been…excluded from school….Also within this group are individuals who had thoughts of self-harm or suicide, some of whom have acted on these feelings" (p. 221).

These teenagers project an aura of hostility to insulate them from intimacy—hence to protect themselves from the risk of being hurt. They often project a facade of grandiosity to hide feelings of vulnerability and inadequacy. Beneath antagonistic exteriors, however, these kids have tender, battered, bruised, and bloodied psyches. They feign apathy, but fear rejection and failure. They exist in a self-imposed hell furnished with the frustration, failure, pain, fear, and rejection which result from their impulsive and poor conscious choices. These feelings of animosity often are caused by fear of being abandoned and betrayed, so they act impulsively to reject before being rejected.

Students at JDA are gifted youngsters whose intellectual, affective, and artistic needs are being ignored. Thus, they act out against an environment they feel is hostile, sterile, and pessimistic by engaging in dangerous and destructive behavior. The presenting problem, reduced to its lowest common dominator, is simply a negative attitude. All experience an identity crisis, which Erikson (1968) describes as follows:

> a…disturbance in…conflicted young people whose sense of confusion is due, rather, to a war within themselves, and in confused rebels and destructive adolescents who war on…society….These new identifications are no longer characterized by the playfulness of childhood and the experimental zest of youth: with dire urgency they force the young individual into choices and decisions which will, with increasing immediacy, lead to commitments "for life" (pp. 17, 155).

Almost two decades later, Wood (1986) agrees with Erikson:

> They do not like themselves and feel angry and impotent at their failure to enjoy life. From this… lack of self-respect, all else stems. They resort to… cunning schemes…to hide…their felt worthlessness….Or, encouraged by psychoanalytic-type philosophies, they blame families,…friends,… circumstances [for their failures]. These individuals are characterized by the "if only" syndrome: "if only things had been different" if only my parents had not… divorced …." "if only I had been born more intelligent, with more money, taller, more attractive," etc. … They shrink from challenges that they feel may put at risk their fragile self-respect …But in attempting to insure against failure by erecting obstacles to success, they make failure more likely and paradoxically the effect is to reduce self-respect…by blaming others, but whatever happens,

the guilt mechanism is not deceived and is never effectively suppressed, causing constant psychological pain" (pp. 15–16).

These youth have abused their intellectual and creative talents. They remain action-oriented to ameliorate agonizing feelings of emptiness and depression. Most Dewey students suffer from what Breggin (1991) has labeled a "psychospiritual crisis" (p. 46).

We have noted several trends during the twenty-two-year history of the John Dewey Academy, trends that parallel our society. For example, the rate of diagnosis of bipolar affective disorder in children and adolescents has exploded during the past five to ten years. Parents arrive at Dewey terrified that the removal of so-called mood stabilizers will precipitate a manic episode. We believe the actual incidence of true bipolar affective disorder is not increasing. It is simply the diagnosis du jour, in much the same way that ADHD was during the 1980s.

Toward a treatment philosophy: A humanistic and pragmatic view

Persons are born with the capacity not only to hope but also to seek meaning. Adolescents need to establish stable personal identities as they learn how to form positive and responsible interpersonal relationships. Until convinced that education is relevant and that learning can be gratifying, these students refuse to invest academically. The classroom teacher thus assumes the burden of convincing them. These angry adolescents need treatment that will force them to accept responsibility for behavior while concurrently helping them recognize the correlation between current acts and future outcomes. The treatment goal is to provide strategies and solutions to change the prognosis from pessimistic to guardedly optimistic. Negative passion needs to be directed into constructive and creative acts.

The therapeutic goal is to nurture the psychological, moral, and spiritual growth of students by creating the conditions conducive to the restoration of self-respect and integrity. Each student has a primary counselor whose caseload rarely exceeds thirteen students. Group therapy is the primary therapeutic approach. Not only does the group insist that the members accept responsibility for self-destructive behavior, it also helps to resolve intrapsychic and interpersonal problems. There are at least four two-hour groups per week, conducted by credentialed therapists with whom the adolescent can relate and peers with whom they can identify. The peers offer insight and suggestions that provide the catalytic conditions necessary for self-exploration and change. Approximately one third of the time is devoted to therapeutic interventions. In addition, students participate nightly in a one-hour self-help group.

In a group setting, students can relate to peers who will confront destructive attitudes while providing catalytic conditions for self-exploration and change. The group demands that members accept responsibility for past failures, and it also helps members to resolve intrapsychic and interpersonal problems. The treatment approach, described more fully in a separate chapter in this volume, utilizes confrontational psychotherapeutic techniques with escalating expectations for improved behavior. Peers confront each other and demand rejection for immature, irresponsible, illicit, and self-destructive acts.

Family members must renegotiate their relationships with the student and with each other. Thus, parental and family involvement is an important component of a JDA stay. Our ultimate mission regarding the family is to help members support the efforts of the John Dewey student to help him/herself. Family therapy sessions, held on weekends when parents are available, focus on changing dysfunctional and dishonest communication patterns. At least eight times a year, parents participate in three two-hour group experiences. In the first group, the parents introduce themselves and discuss their concerns. In the second group, which is intergenerational in nature, members are separated so that they will elicit help from others. The third group is a mothers and fathers group where discussion focuses on role-related problems. When there are sufficient siblings, there is a brothers and sisters group.

Institutional aspects of JDA

Despite JDA's efforts not to be "institutional," it is an institution. For a minimum of eighteen months, students live a safe, womb-like nurturing environment. As in colleges, the military, hospitals, and jails, our students do not have to worry about survival issues such as food, clothing, and shelter. Students receive a nominal weekly allowance to help them learn the value of money, and how to manage it.

Biological reductionism: Counter therapeutic to growth

Our opposition to medication is based on our belief that viewing problems as being caused by metabolic disorders, genetic imbalances, and cellular deficiencies is not helpful for the treatment of these youngsters. No pill teaches self-respect or cures noxious narcissism, deceit, and antisocial attitudes.

A focus on symptoms, rather than understanding the adolescent's world view, ignores the crucial information that is necessary for understanding etiology. Removing the symptoms, without addressing behavioral and attitude, compounds the problem because it breeds impotence and dejection. Worse, this reductionistic thinking reinforces excuses for poor choices and continuing negative behaviors.

Prescribing psychotropic medication transmits a counter therapeutic message—i.e., adolescents cannot cope and do not need to try. The attribution of depression to a chemical imbalance has spawned a proliferation of psychopharmacological treatment, and its advocates, whose views are exemplified by Koplewicz (2002) when he writes:

> Medicine should be prescribed carefully and deliberately. Unfortunately, there is an almost universal belief by the public that teenagers should first try psychotherapy, and medication should be considered only after

that fails. This idea comes from two mistaken and outdated beliefs: 1) that medications may be addictive or dangerous to teenagers, and 2) that depression in young people is caused either by early trauma or by some intrinsic weakness in the teenager that can be overcome with psychotherapy (p. 262).

The readiness to resort to medication stems from the search for a quick fix and from the therapist's sense of impotence. At the very least, concerns on the part of regulatory agencies about the safety of antidepressant medications in children and adolescents should lead to greater caution in their use. The over-emphasis on biological aspects of depression ignores the impact of toxic acts, conscious attitudes, and personal choice.

Whittington et al. (2004) warn, in their systematic review of published and unpublished studies of serotonin reuptake inhibitor drugs:

> In view of the high risk of suicide in this group of children and young people, the possibility that a drug might increase that risk without clear evidence of benefit should, in our view, discourage its use….A possible increased risk of suicidal ideation, serious adverse events, or both, although small, cannot be ignored (p. 1344).

Finally, most adolescents in our program report that they feel more alert and energetic when they are taken off medication.

Diagnosing: A counter therapeutic activity?

Lack of reliability

In today's climate of third-party payers and dependence on the biological quick fix, diagnostic interviews are often unreliable. This is not a new problem, but it is a worsening one. A senior staff psychologist at the Menninger Foundation, Applebaum (1977) asserts that "diagnosing…is a hyperabstract… intellectual exercise associated with a loss of feeling toward and emotional contact with a patient" (p. 161). Confirming Applebaum, Maxmen and Ward (1995) suggest that the differential diagnosis may be more subjective than generally acknowledged.

Diagnosing the psychosocial characteristics of deceitful, drug-dependent adolescents is an even more complex matter. The interviewer lacks the time (and often the skill) to establish a therapeutic alliance with the adolescent, so the youth remains guarded and dishonest. Exacerbating this problem is that these youngsters are sophisticated, so they manipulate the clinician, viewed as the enemy, with ease.

A DSM-IV diagnosis inadvertently provides justification and excuses for poor behavior. In our experience, many addicted adolescents often welcome these diagnoses as excuses for their behavior—and as justification for the prescription of psychotropic medication. These drugs can be used inappropriately, or can be sold on the black market.

Problems with labeling

Sperry (1995) warns about the consequences of labeling:

> Mention personality disorders—particularly borderline personality disorder or antisocial disorder—to a colleague and you might elicit such comments as, "Most borderlines are treatment refractory," "Personality disorders have guarded prognoses at best," or "Antisocial (persons) are psychopaths and should be in prison, not psychotherapy." And what about your reaction when a colleague wants to refer a personality disordered individual to you. Do you feel stuck, apprehensive, or angry? Do you think about your…safety, after-hours emergencies or telephone calls, and whether your bill will be paid? (p. 1).

Diagnostic labeling leads to lowered expectations by the therapist, which allows the youth to settle for mediocrity. Program philosophy and treatment outcome, furthermore, will be adversely affected by negative and positive self-fulfilling prophesies related to the diagnosis. Verbalizing these concerns, Meeks (1989) cautions:

> We need to remember the risk of overdiagnosing and overlabeling…From a countertransference point of view, there is…a temptation to overdiagnose… abrasive or hostile adolescents. The angry therapist can say, "I am beginning to feel that this youngster has a psychotic (or paranoid) core." Translation: "This adolescent does not like me nearly as much as he/she should, considering what a good therapist I am" (p. 3).

Making an accurate DSM-IV diagnosis is further complicated by the effects of psychoactive substances that can mimic symptoms of psychosis and/or depression. Amphetamines can cause a temporary psychotic state and can also induce a condition resembling hypomania. Marijuana and amphetamines can both produce paranoid symptoms. Opiates and marijuana can induce apathetic states consistent with major depressive disorder. In addition, drug abuse wreaks havoc on sleep and appetite patterns, further complicating the diagnostic picture. Weiss and Millman (1991) contend that psychotic disorders, occurring subsequent to prolonged drug use, can be manifestations of premorbid psychopathology. Greene (1996) urges prudent precautions prior to diagnosis. Clinicians need to take into account the acute and chronic impacts of drug abuse. Definitive diagnosis must wait until detoxification in order to ascertain which symptoms relate directly to the drug use, and which predate it.

The diagnostic process, as Pruyser and Menninger (1976) note, can be influenced by value judgments reflecting the orientation and bias of the mental health worker:

> Upon reading psychiatric reports, one is struck by tendencies which, for many writers, have become habits....Moralization comes through in such words as perversion, psychopathic, inadequate personality, infantile personality, and character disorder. Outright accusatory expressions are castrating female, passive father, and schizophrenogenic mother. Some word usage substitutes perjorative meanings: compulsive for orderly, depressed for sad (p. 25).

Szasz (1961), using incendiary rhetoric, makes the valid point that what masquerades for a diagnosis often reflects the bias of the therapist (and institution), thus justifying the prescription of medication. The use of psychiatric nomenclature in order to receive third-party payments is now de rigeur. This article is a plea never to forget that patients remain people who have intentionally hurt themselves and others.

What was normal then is abnormal now

Changes in normative behavior have called into question the validity of some diagnostic criteria. Before the 1960s, distinguishing between normal and abnormal was less complicated than it is today. At the beginning of the 1960s, drug use and early sexual activity fell outside the norm. In the 21st century, the distinction between responsible and irresponsible has become blurred. Testing limits, questioning and/or rejecting authority, have become the norm. The blurring of absolutes renders assessment more subjective because it is more contaminated by the diagnostician's values and experience.

In the third millennium, experimentation with drugs and sex has become the primary rite of initiation into adolescence. When discussing the oral sex epidemic of the 1990s, which has become pandemic during the third millennium, Dennis (1992), a female Canadian journalist, writes:

> While having a [female] on her knees is by no means a prerequisite for a splendiferous blowjob, for some [males] it is the penultimate erotic charge. That's because with a [female] on her knees, a [male] can imagine all kinds of nasty, lovely power associations. (...Coming in a [female's] mouth, doing her up the bun or doggie-style gives many [males] a glowy feeling.)

The kneeling business, however, has sparked a passionate debate about whether there's such a thing as a politically correct blowjob, and it goes straight to the heart of one of the most controversial issues of sexual politics of our time. Some [females] agonize whether they should agree to perform blowjobs in a kneeling position (or do that other submissive stuff lots of guys seem to love) because complying means assuming blatantly servile postures, and we...know how [females] feel on that subject. What drives [females] completely nutso on this volatile matter, however, is the fact that a fair number of them…get their *own* erotic buzz from performing the handmaiden role in these little fantasy-dramas (p. 162).

Incredibly, those who abstain are in the minority—hence, different. "Well-adjusted" adolescents can write dark poetry, can play and listen to gloomy music, can glorify celebrities who committed suicide or died of drug overdoses, can fantasize about aberrant acts, periodically dramatically scream, cry, and threaten suicide. However, they do not become addicted to psychoactive substances, self-mutilate in frankly self destructive ways, develop eating disorders, or commit violent acts. Whitaker (1989) laments:

> Teenagers who don't drink (the most popular American drug is alcohol) often must make plans to conceal their abstinence while so-called "normal" teenagers line their rooms with empty liquor bottles and beer ads and go around advertising beer on T-shirts that generally cost twice as much as highest cotton T-shirts unadorned with other people's commercial ploys. The success of these ploys show the genius of advertisers; advertisers have actually gotten customers to pay the alcohol industry and their advertisers a premium for plugging alcohol. Mark Twain's Tom Sawyer, who got a boy to whitewash a fence by touting that work is a privilege, has been one-upped by the alcohol industry (p. 25).

Changes in adolescence demand new treatment approaches

Developments such as those described in the preceding section present new challenges for therapists. Friedman (1991) warns "the perils of adolescence as a developmental stage have been increased during the past decade" (p. 363), thus necessitating a more active-directive treatment approach. The mass media has extolled "drug usage, sexual freedom, … and an anti-work ethic" (p. 364). Many adolescents engage in dangerous behaviors from which they are unable to extricate themselves.

> They cannot navigate between the Scylla of excessive rigidity and the Charybdis of passive gratification. For them, effective psychotherapy requires a therapist who is willing to help them develop skills in navigation by recognizing the dangers from both sides….The therapist may have to stand firm against such influence with adolescent patients. He may have to do so with vigor and force when the adolescent's inner life is enforced by authority figures who define autonomy in passive, regressive fashions (pp. 364, 365).

Another approach

We contend that pathological beliefs and dysfunctional behaviors can be changed. We agree with Breggin (1991), who states, "By refusing to diagnose or to label people who already feel rejected and humiliated, we welcome them back to the human community and promote humane, respectful, and loving attitudes toward them" (p. 46). As do Mowrer (1961), Ellis (1962), and Glasser (1965), we reject the psychoanalytic approach because we believe that focusing on learning and growth in the present are key aspects of a successful treatment. Adolescents can transcend their pasts. As Patterson et al. (2005) propose, the individual "cannot...control conditions [by] which he is confronted. but can control his responses....[The person] is responsible for his responses, his choices, and his actions" (p. 466). Another way is to look at depression as a realistic response to self-destructive behavior.

As we have indicated, most entering students arrive with multiple psychiatric diagnoses, most often including a depressive spectrum disorder. Depression, common during adolescence, can be a product of self-destructive behavior and antisocial attitudes, which lead to "self-criticism, self-contempt, self-deprecation, self-doubt, self-punishment...seeing the worst in [one's self]; by...low self-esteem; and by accompanying feelings of failure, inadequacy, worthlessness, embarrassment, guilt" (Driscoll, 1989, p. 104). Driscoll fails to note that poor conscious choices are at the root of this teenage malaise. In addition to decreasing future options, these adolescents have destroyed relationships with family and friends. They feel, as a result, alone and betrayed. They trust no one. While they are indeed depressed, their problems cannot be cured with medication.

Between clinical depression, attributed to a metabolic deficiency, and reality-based despair exists a profound difference, although the surface symptoms may be quite similar. Kids know they have compromised their futures, so depression is a realistic reaction. When asked why they feel depressed, gifted adolescents can articulate and provide substantial, realistic explanations. Due to poor conscious decisions, they have imprisoned themselves in a lose-lose labyrinth. Thus begins the cycle of hopelessness, helplessness, and demoralization—hardly prerequisites for constructive and creative change. These adolescents believe they are damaged goods. They stop daring to dream that they can rebuild their lives, thus intensifying their despair. Is it any wonder they resemble patients with mood disorders?

Converting anger and shame into proactive behavior: A treatment challenge

Viewed in this light, the primary cause of depression is a toxic, self-induced attitude that is compounded and perpetuated by dysfunctional behavior, resulting in feelings of pain, shame, fear, inadequacy, and self-loathing. Underneath the thin layer of depression exists an intense rage. The sources of this rage are voracious entitlement needs, a self-serving sense of injustice, and a full retreat into the role of the victim. The clinical challenge is to redirect this anger/rage into positive, productive, and proactive activities. Gans & Weber (2000) contend "shame is an important emotion that… [group] leaders…overlook, often to the detriment of their groups.… Attention to shame requires clinical judgment, proper timing, countertransference awareness, and a primary obligation to the needs of the members of the group" (pp. 393, 394). Nathanson (1987) discusses the centrality of shame in adolescent development. Kaufman (1989) asserts, "no other affect is more disturbing to the self, none more central for the sense of identity. In the context of normal development, shame is the source of low self-esteem, diminished self-image, poor self-concept.…Shame…produces self-doubts and disrupts… security and confidence" (p. vii). Helping students recognize that guilt and shame result from irresponsible and/or illicit acts is an effective treatment tactic, because this pain creates the incentive to change.

It can be salubrious when the therapist states, "I understand why you suffer, because what you did is hurtful and hateful. If you change your behavior, you will feel better about yourself." An intense group experience forces these adolescents toward accountability and also toward a true comprehension of the correlation between current acts and attitudes and outcomes and consequences. The clinical challenge is to help adolescents ameliorate noxious feelings by discovering positive behavioral options. When behavior becomes congruent with a positive value system, adolescents gain self-respect. In contrast, we note that sympathy can prolong the homeostasis which mires individuals in self-imposed depressive states.

Restoration of hope: The most potent cure for depression

To ameliorate despair, the teenager needs to be convinced that change is possible. Adolescents arrive at Dewey demoralized because they know their acts have destroyed future options. A significant number have refused to study since elementary school, and have even been school avoidant. Of course, it is impossible to hide from the transcript, a black and white confrontation in and of itself. These students lack the incentive to work because they know the best they can do is a fourth-or fifth-rate college. We believe that until the student feels there is a modicum of hope that the future can indeed improve, the person will not study. Hope, therefore, becomes the primary catalyst for change.

During the intake interview, the applicant is told that all our graduates attend college and most are accepted by the most competitive institutions of higher learning. Outside the president's office where the interview occurs, are two plaques which contain the names of graduates and the colleges they attended. Alexander & French (1946) note:

> Like the adage, nothing succeeds like success, there is no more powerful therapeutic factor than the performance of activities.…No insight, no

emotional discharge, and no recollection can be as reassuring as accomplishment in the actual life experience in which the individual has failed. Thus the ego regains that confidence which is the fundamental condition, the prerequisite of mental health. Every success encourages new trials, and decreases inferiority feelings....*Successful attempts at productive work, love, self-assertion, or competition will change the vicious cycle to begin one; as they are repeated, they become habitual and thus eventually bring about a complete change in the personality* (p. 40, italics added).

Elsewhere in this volume, Bratter discusses the power of the impact that the therapeutic act of advocacy has on the restoration of hope.

Life after JDA

Graduation from high school, in our society, starts the transition to young adulthood. High school seniors enjoy status and security and may thus be a bit reluctant to close the final chapter of adolescence. For most adolescents, going to college is exciting but also frightening and threatening, because it means starting again, being at the bottom, and knowing no one.

JDA seniors participate in a year-long weekly senior group that maximizes the probability of success. By this time the members have participated in approximately 1,000 hours in other groups, so they know each other well. Our senior experience is divided into five sequential components: a) bonding with classmates to build a support network after graduation; b) coping with pressures of confronting peers to improve themselves, thus encouraging the internalization of proactive values; c) becoming moral leaders and responsible role models; d) training juniors to assume positive leadership roles and saying good-bye to them; and e) gaining the courage of convictions to resist the myriad of self-destructive activities at college. Students discuss and ponder real issues such as, "What do I say if my roommate wants to use the room as either a brothel or drug den?" This decreases significantly the probability of becoming a casualty or dropout.

Outcome data

The dropout rate from JDA since its inception is less than twenty-five percent. If a student chooses to leave, the school works with the family to find the adolescent another residential program, because the school is committed to forcing the student to "grow up."

Table 7.1 shows a list of the colleges attended by JDA graduates. More than seventy percent of JDA graduates graduate from college. More than a third make the dean's list at college. At least a third attend graduate school. Ten percent are either attending or have graduated from law schools. In the new millennium, less than ten percent of Dewey graduates have dropped out. Equally significant, less

Table 7.1   Colleges John Dewey Academy graduates have attended

Antioch College	Grinnell College*	Spelman College*
Babson College*	Hamilton College	St. John's College
Barnard College*	Hampshire College	SUNY-Binghampton
Bates College*	Haverford College*	SUNY-Purchase
Bennington College	Hobart College*	Syracuse University*
Bentley College	Indiana University	College of Visual Arts,
Berkshire Community	Kalamazoo College	Martin J. Whitman School
College*	Kenyon College	of International
Boston College	Lemoyne College	Management, S.I.
Boston University	Manhattanville College	Newhouse School of
Brandeis University	Mary Washington	Public Communication
Brown University*	University	Trinity College*
Bucknell University*	Mount Holyoke College*	Tufts University*
Carleton College*	Muhlenberg College*	Tulane University
Clark University	New York University Tisch	Union College*
Centre College	School of Arts*	UCLA
College of the Holy Cross*	Northwestern University	University of Chicago*
Columbia College*	Oberlin College*	University of Hartford*
Columbia University*	Ohio Wesleyan University*	University of Hawaii
Connecticut College*	Parsons School of Design	University of
Cornell University*	Pepperdine University	Massachusetts*
Eckert College	Pitzer College	University of Miami
Embry Riddle Aeronautical	Queens University	University of Michigan
University	(Canada)	(Honors Program)
Emerson College	Rollins College	University of Oregon*
George Washington	Rensselaer Polytechnic	University of Rochester*
University*	Institute*	University of Santa Clara
Georgetown University*	Sarah Lawrence College	University of Tampa
Glendon College of the	Scripps College	University of the Redlands
University of Toronto	Skidmore College*	Vassar College*
(Canada)		Wellesley College*
		Wheaton College
		Williams College*

*   Denotes Dean's List

than ten percent of this school's alumni resume psychotherapy or take psychotropic medication as adults.

Both interesting and significant is the fact that there is little staff turnover. Most staff members have doctorates. A majority of the faculty have been at the school for at least a decade.

Conclusion

In summary, the John Dewey Academy provides a positive educational and emotional experience that promotes:

- Maximizing the making of constructive and creative choices
- Formulating realistic intermediate to long-term educational, personal, and professional goals and the strength to achieve them
- Individuation and separation from the family
- A proactive self-identity
- Forming mature and positive interpersonal relationships
- Strength to be assertive and moral
- The opportunity to (re)gain self-respect
- The incentive to be good and decent
- A resilience to learn and survive inevitable painful fears, failure, and rejection
- An optimistic outlook about one's self and capacity to succeed at tasks considered important
- A desire to change rather than remain complacent
- The ability to take control of one's life by making conscious, responsible, and proactive choices
- The courage to shatter restricting boundaries of innocence and ignorance which characterize immature thinking

Given the energy, enthusiasm, and creativity of adolescents who yearn for novelty, self-destructive acts may signal the "rites" of passage from childhood to adolescence in our society. The nature of this rebellion changes for each generation, but teens still seek personal identities, and they still battle their conflicting needs between desire for the security of dependence and the struggle for independence and separation from the family. Youth continue to rebel by hurting themselves and those who love them. When convinced it is in their best interest, however, they work diligently to achieve success at those tasks they consider important and stimulating.

References

Alexander, F. & French, T. (1946), *Psychoanalytic Therapy*. New York: Ronald Press.

Applebaum, S. A. (1977), Objections to diagnostic psychological testing. In *Diagnosis and the Difference It Makes*, ed. P. W. Pruyser, New York: Jason Aronson, pp. 161–174.

Bratter, T. E., Bratter, C. J., Maxym, C., & Steiner, K.S. (1998), The John Dewey Academy, a moral caring community: An amalgamation of the professional model and self-help concept of the therapeutic community. In *Community as Method: Modified Therapeutic Communities for Special Populations and Special Settings*, eds. G. De Leon, & J. F. Zeingfus. Westport, CT: Greenwood Publishers, pp. 179–194.

Breggin, P. (1991), *Toxic Psychiatry: Why Therapy, Empathy, and Love Must Replace the Drugs, Electroshock, and Biochemical Theories of the New Psychiatry*. New York: St. Martin's Press.

Dennis, W. (1992), *Hot and Bothered: Sex & Love in the Nineties*. New York: Viking Press.

Ellis, A. (1962), *Reason and Emotion in Psychotherapy*. New York: Lyle Stuart.

Friedman, H. (1991), Confrontation in the psychotherapy of adolescent patients. In: *Confrontation in Psychotherapy*, ed. G. Adler & P. G. Myerson. Northvale, NJ: Jason Aronson, pp. 349–367.

Gans, J. S., & Weber, R. L. (2000), The detection of shame in group psychotherapy: Uncovering the hidden emotion. *Intl. J. Group Psychother.*, 50:381–396.

Giddens, A. (1991), *Modernity and Self Identity.* Stanford, CA: Stanford University Press.

Glasser, W., (1965), *Reality Therapy: A New Approach to Psychiatry.* New York: Harper & Row.

Harris, J. (2005), The increased diagnosis of "juvenile bipolar disorder": What are we treating? *Psychiat. Serv.*, 56:529–531.

Kaufman, G. (1989), *The Psychology of Shame: Theory and Treatment of Shame-Based Syndromes.* New York: Springer.

Meeks, J. E. (1989), Diagnosis and psychotherapy of adolescents. *Highland Highlights* 2:2–6.

Mowrer, O. H. (1961), *The Crisis in Psychiatry and Religion.* Princeton, NJ: D. Van Nostrand.

Nathanson, D. (1987), *The Many Faces of Shame.* New York: Guilford.

Patterson, K., Grenny, J., McMillan, R., & Switzer, A. (2005), *Crucial Confrontations: Tools for Resolving Broken Promises, Violated Expectations, and Bad Behavior.* New York: McGraw-Hill.

Pruyser, P. W. & Menninger K. (1976), Language pitfalls in diagnostic thought and work. In: *Diagnosis and the Difference it Makes*, ed. P. W. Pruyser. New York: Jason Aronson, pp. 11–28.

Rose, J. (2004), The residential care and treatment of adolescents. In *From Toxic Institutions to Therapeutic Environments: Residential Settings in Mental Health Services*, ed. P. Campling, S. Davies, & G. Farquharson. Gaskell, UK: Royal College of Psychiatrists, pp. 219–226.

Sperry, L. (1995), *Handbook of Diagnosis and Treatment of the DSM-IV Personality Disorders.* New York: Brunner/Mazel.

Szasz, T. S. (1961), *The Myth of Mental Illness: Foundations of a Theory of Personal Conduct.* New York: Harper.

Whittington, C. J., Kendall, T., Fonagy, P., Cottrell, D., Citgrove, A., & Boddington, E. (2004), Selective serotonin reuptake inhibitors in childhood depression: Systematic review of published versus unpublished data. *Lancet,* 369:1341–1345.

8 Advocacy

Its impact on the treatment alliance with gifted, self-destructive, and drug-abusing adolescents

Thomas Edward Bratter

Abstract

This article is a plea to therapists, especially those who work with gifted, dysfunctional, and disenfranchised adolescents, to add advocacy to their armamentarium. These adolescents resist forming a therapeutic alliance, but they know they have compromised their educational and professional options. The most effective way to connect with them is to offer to be an advocate for them. This involves becoming a power broker to plead for a favorable outcome with authorities who have the power to grant or refuse the adolescent's access to upward mobility. The population described in this chapter remains immune to traditional psychotherapy, and indeed must be engaged quickly in therapy for success to occur. If the therapist fails to discuss his or her intention to work for the adolescent's best interests at the outset, the adolescent probably will not return for a second session. The actual advocacy efforts are made after the adolescent fulfills his or her part of the contract. Although this chapter will focus on advocacy in the college admissions process, advocacy can encompass other proactive activities: to convince an employer to hire, to persuade a family member or a friend to reconcile, to intervene in criminal proceedings by suggesting alternatives to incarceration, to secure housing, and so on.

Advocacy: A treatment innovation

Little has been written about the psychotherapist as advocate and about the impact of advocacy on the therapeutic alliance with adolescents. Indeed, Masterson (1989a) bemoans that his magnum opus on adolescence, *Treatment of the Borderline Adolescent* (1972), "was greeted with thundering silence" (p. xv). When reviewing advocacy, Myers, Sweeney, and White (2002) lament "a review of the literature in counseling…revealed few sources on advocacy for the profession" (p. 394). Eriksen (1997) observes that "no one has researched advocacy [for] the counseling field" (p. 2).

Agreeing with Stone (1971), I (Bratter, 1977) describe advocacy as "a unique relationship in which the psychotherapist…attempts to gain preferential consideration for [persons in treatment]" (p. 121). Vash (1987) exhorts rehabilitation professionals to recognize that advocacy is a counseling imperative, but provides no therapeutic strategies.

Advocacy can favorably impact outcomes with various treatment populations, but it is essential when working with youth who do not respond to traditional psychotherapies—a group that includes many adolescents (Meeks and Bernet, 1990). Freud excluded persons in crisis from psychoanalysis. Acting-out adolescents create perpetual crises to which the therapist must respond, thus making an analytically oriented approach difficult.

Aichhorn (1935) warns "dissocial children do not come to us of their...free will but are brought to us [against their desires]. To the dissocial child we are a menace because we represent society, with which he is in conflict....It is hard to make some of these delinquent children talk. One thing they...have in common; they do not tell the truth" (p. 124). Aichhorn (1964) further notes that the burden to convince the teenager to return for the second session remains that of the therapist:

> Most juvenile delinquents meet us at first with utter distrust and their suspicions must be swiftly overcome before we can win them over. Such suspiciousness is not...pathological; the child guidance worker appears as something dangerous to him....In keeping with the unpleasant experiences he has had so far with adults, he is entitled to expect something distasteful....He therefore feels immediately compelled to consider the personality of the counselor (p. 158).

As Hanna, Hanna, and Keyes have noted, gifted and alienated teenagers are defiant, suspicious, hostile, and resistant to therapy (1999). Despite Meeks and Bernet's (1990) attempt to modify psychoanalytic technique to include more types of adolescents, they are wrong to suggest that "effective confrontation... [shows] the patient what he is doing either without knowing it or without recognizing its importance" (pp. 163, 162). Perhaps this is the reason they are forced to acknowledge that some teenagers are untreatable. They state, "If the patient's mistrust of others, defensive structure, or living situation makes an alliance impossible, it is preferable to admit that and suggest termination" (1990, p. 287). Giovacchini (1985) believes adolescents possess a "propensity for creating problems within the treatment setting because of their reticence about becoming engaged, or their inclination to express themselves through action rather than words and feelings" (p. 447). Katz (1998) concludes "the establishment of the therapeutic alliance is one of the major...challenges faced by adolescent psychiatrists" (p. 89).

My position is that the therapist's offering to be an advocate may be the crucial link to forming a therapeutic alliance and, thus, to treatability. If the student rejects the therapist's offer to be an advocate (or refuses to make a commitment to change—part of the advocacy agreement), and assuming the risk of self-destructive behavior is extreme, the psychotherapist may need to consider residential treatment.

Even if these youngsters return for a second session, their problems persist. Countertransference and transference can become major obstacles to effective therapy. The psychotherapist can use an idealizing tranference to build the treatment alliance by stating that the adolescent can excel and that such excellence will make the advocate's "mission impossible" easier. Early in treatment, I do not discourage idealization of the therapist. However, these feelings must be terminated so the student can become assertive and autonomous. Meeks and Bernet (1990), rightfully so, warn that omnipotent transference can be seductive but it impedes growth because it nurtures dependence.

> The expectation that the therapist has answers...and solutions...bears enough similarity to some ordinary, or at least fantasized, relationships between the generations to be quite attractive....It is easy to drift gradually into a relationship in which the adolescent presents as a helpless, idiotic emotional cripple, repeatedly rescued from disaster only because of the brilliance of the therapist....As gratifying as such a situation may be to the therapist's narcissism and his infantile omnipotence, it is catastrophic to the goals of psychotherapy (p. 175).

The treatment goal is to create the conditions for helping the adolescent to individuate and separate from the family and therapist, and to become a mature individual who defines goals and wants to fulfill personal needs.

As Nagel (1989) points out, "acting-out behaviors can be disturbing to therapists and trigger countertransference feelings. The therapist may act out with the patient by becoming angry, attacking, or withdrawing.... Out of frustration, therapists may use interpretation to deal with their *own* [italics in the original] feelings...." (pp. 405–406).

Drug-abusing teens know that self-medication can provide temporary relief and, unless the psychotherapist assumes an active-directive approach, they will continue to abuse psychoactive substances. Amodeo and Drouilhet (1992) caution "therapists working with adolescents who use dangerous...drugs must examine their...values, attitudes, and visceral reactions to these patients....Some clinicians will struggle with feelings of moralism, anger, or anxiety... but in the end may realize that they will never be effective with this population" (p. 305).

Advocacy and the restoration of hope

The therapist's promise to intervene restores hope for future outcomes which, in turn, provides incentive for the adolescent to enter into a therapeutic transaction. The therapist needs to persuade the teenager to start a treatment relationship by reassuring the youth that success can be achieved when he or she works diligently. "Why," I ask the youth, "would I invest so much energy if I did not think you can succeed and are worth my effort?" By making poor choices, self-destructive adolescents have trapped themselves in a lose-lose labyrinth in which frustration, fear, rejection, and failure become negative and painful self-fulfilling prophecies. Alienated students have lost hope because they feel impotent to escape from a self-imposed plight. Dejection is a realistic reaction to an environment that unconvinced juveniles feel is too pessimistic to endure. When the psychotherapist communicates "you cannot" rather than "you can," the impact on the therapeutic dyad is debilitating. The therapist who urges the youngster to reduce educational and personal goals essentially concedes defeat. Who wants to be a loser (or work with one)? Horney (1945) describes the corrosive impact of hopelessness and implores the psychoanalyst to communicate optimistic expectations. Frankl's existential view is particularly germane to the adolescent phase of life—"If we take man as he is, we make him worse; if we take him as he ought to be, we help him become it" (1967, p. 27).

There is abundant evidence from psychiatric and nonpsychiatric medicine to indicate that hope affects outcome. Oncologists know the difference between patients who have quit and those who retain the will to live. When patients feel they can surmount physical ailments, they are more likely to succeed than are those who refuse to try (Thompson, Soboloaw-Shubin, Galbraith, Schwankvosky, & Druzen, 1993; Petersen, 2000; Taylor, Kenneny, Reed, Bower, & Greenwald, 2003). Alexander (1962) asserts that "a change from a state of hopelessness to hopeful expectation revitalizes the integrative powers of the ego, which then reactivate the active personality" (p. 174). Armor and Taylor (1998) confirm that the restoration of hope is a potent curative force for self-betterment. Stotland (1969) suggests the "greater the expectation of attaining a goal, the more likely the individual will...attain it" (p. 17).

Advocacy in psychotherapy

Many youth, who are not amenable to traditional therapy, do respond positively to a treatment dyad motto of "us against the world." The advocate-psychotherapist becomes what Blos (1962) has termed a "special friend" (and, perhaps, an idealized parent). With each success, the teenager invests more in improvement, thus decreases resistance and regression. This dynamic can change when necessary to challenge and confront illicit and destructive acts. This transformation shifts the therapist (from the adolescent's perspective) into the critical parent/superego introject.

Fostering personal responsibility

Thirty years ago, I learned that when becoming an aggressive advocate, I could help the teenager (re)gain self-respect. My colleagues and I (Bratter, Bratter, & Bratter, 1995) have contended that this is the ultimate goal of therapy. Helping the adolescent to accept responsibility and accountability remains quintessential to the psychotherapeutic process.

The therapist needs to convince a skeptical youth about the long-term benefits of change. Acceptance by and graduation from a college of quality closes the door on a painful past. Davis and Paster (2000) propose that the establishment of a mentor relationship helps the adolescent develop resiliency and optimism. Luthar and Zigler (1991) and Garmezy and Rutter (1983) confirm that a resilient child often can identify one adult who has taken a special interest. Such external validation restores hope that growth and success are realistic objectives. Advocacy places the psychotherapist in a charismatic role as a problem-solver–consultant-coach. Williams and Davis (2002) write, "Coaches aid clients in creating visions and goals for all aspects of their lives and in creating multiple strategies to support those goals" (pp. xiv-xv). When the adolescent begins to dare to dream about success, the probability of a positive outcome increases. The psychotherapist's becoming an advocate has a salutary impact on the restoration of morale, which enables the professional to maintain high expectations for improved behavior performance" (Bratter, 1977). I negotiate a quid-pro-quo agreement that is held in abeyance until the student changes. The statement "*after* you do what you need to do, then I'll help you achieve your goals" generates the leverage to demand improved performance.

My praise "to your credit, you have improved" not only reinforces empowerment but also communicates an expectation to improve. I do not respond, "I am proud of you"; that comment implies possessiveness, which can provoke a negative transference-countertransference response. Instead, I state "I'm happy for you," thus giving credit to the adolescent for diligent work.

I do not guarantee that my efforts will be successful. This promise strengthens the treatment alliance because the student (and/or family) view me as an asset who can play a critical role to help them achieve a valued outcome. If the youth and parents verbalize appreciation, I emphasize the student's performance. I acknowledge that my letter helped achieve a positive outcome but I assert "all I did was to describe your son's or daughter's behavior. The kid did the work." A dean of admission once wrote, "You write the most amazing recommendations I have ever read! Truly incredible! I appreciated Matthew's honest personal statement, as well as your helpful recommendation. My question, given no visit here, is whether you can shed any light on what the late application means. Are we are a distant choice?" Since the applicant used this college as a "safety," I advised the dean that Matthew be placed on the waiting list which would not penalize the college for admitting a student who would not attend since the acceptance-attendance ratio often determines status. I did not discuss this correspondence with the student or the family.

The college admissions process

Selective colleges can fill first-year classes multiple times without compromising standards. College admissions never have been more competitive. Even academic excellence, high standardized test scores, impressive extracurricular activities, and superlative recommendations no longer guarantee admission to a college of quality. Bratter and Hammerschlag (1975) lament that "many…institutions have become so complicated...that individuals no longer have direct access to them. There are waiting lists, esoteric admissions criteria....Bureaucratic barriers, indeed, are formidable" (p. 128). For the student with a flawed record, the obstacles are daunting. The advocate's task is to convince the committee of admissions to admit this student and in so doing, reject a qualified applicant.

In general, to maximize the chance of admission, noncompetitive applicants need to apply "early decision." The advocate must convince the committee of admissions that the student will attend; otherwise, the office of admissions will be reluctant to invest additional time considering the specialness of the applicant. There are some cases, however, in which the student should decline to apply early decision. Unless at least a one-year relationship exists, the therapist-advocate will have little credibility with the committee of admissions. In addition, if the student has not demonstrated for one year that he or she can excel academically, it would be folly to submit an early decision application. There are unique considerations in advocating for an applicant who has a troubled past. Mediocre academic performance, the least severe form of destructive behavior, cannot be camouflaged in a college application. In contrast, most other forms of dangerous acts—physical scars caused by self-mutilation, abortion, drug abuse, suicide attempts, incarceration, institutionalization, and so on—can be hidden. Confidentiality statutes prohibit disclosure of self-injurious acts and crimes.

When writing an application, the college candidate cannot advocate effectively for him/herself by detailing personal changes; these explanations can appear self-righteous, arrogant, and/or disingenuous. The therapist has more credibility because the advocate possesses the expertise to provide reasonable assurance about the probability of success. The therapist, who is uniquely qualified, can describe the applicant's strengths and weaknesses, depict the humanity of the student, and document proactive changes. A letter of recommendation can be the difference between rejection and acceptance.

The letter of recommendation

A recommendation can resemble a case summary, with the caveat that the therapist should avoid the use of clinical and diagnostic terms. Psychobabble is disconcerting for admissions committees, who lack clinical sophistication. The writer needs to explain how the applicant has emerged from a painful pathological ordeal to become a stronger, more sensitive, and saner individual who has the courage of personal convictions, self-respect, a positive concept of self, plus a commitment to act proactively. The writer should avoid glamorizing hedonistic life styles, but should emphasize that recovering youth are less likely to regress (since they know the shame and pain they caused themselves) than the naive who have not been exposed to the painful verities of life.

I send my recommendation *before* the college interview, so the student can discuss his or her reaction to what I have written, thus partially structuring the interview. (Based on student reports and admissions personnel comments, more than 90% of the recommendations have been read.) A thoughtful recommendation can impress the interviewer since the defiant youth's recovery is interesting and inspirational. In fact, kids who have acted out are often paradoxically alluring, owing to their emancipation from middle-class constraints. Frequently these self-destructive students are more charismatic, articulate, and socially sophisticated than those who have not been initiated into the adolescent counterculture. Most recommendations written by deans, counselors, and teachers are superficial (hence not likely to pique the reader's interest) because these writers do not know much about the applicant and they fear litigation if confidential information is disclosed. Since the applicant's cumulative record is not competitive, the advocate needs to explain to the student and family that acceptance depends on a realistic discussion of extenuating circumstances. A perfunctory letter is irrelevant. Prior to sending the recommendation, I give the candidate a copy to edit. This is to ensure the information is accurate and also to involve the student in the process. I request that the student sign a statement which gives permission to send the letter and releases me from liability.

When the recommendation contains disturbing material, the advocate needs to contact the reader to discuss the letter, answer questions, and provide assurance that the student has grown from painful failures and will become a moral leader, trusted and respected by peers and faculty members. After sending such a letter, the advocate should schedule an on-campus interview with the highest-ranking admissions professional available. If possible, the advocate should accompany the student for the interview because this commitment impresses the admissions counselor. I ask the admissions professional what the applicant can do to be admitted. Surprisingly, this question often is answered. I send a letter to confirm the agreement.

Hallowitz (1974) lists some additional strategies the advocate can use: making phone calls, writing letters, and attending conferences. Grosser (1965) counsels the advocate to be assertive. The advocate needs to understand the differences between assertion, aggression, and abrasiveness. I have contacted the president of the college, dean of admissions, and/or professors to gain support. I have spoken with trustees, alumni, and benefactors and have sent them a copy of my recommendation (with the permission of the student) to urge them to write letters.

An effective recommendation has five primary components: (1) a candid description of the applicant's destructive behavior; (2) an explanation of the candidate's corrective emotional experience; (3) evidence of the adolescent's growth; (4) assurance that the adolescent will improve the quality of life in the classroom and on the campus; and (5) documentation of the writer's expertise. The following recommendation illustrates these points.

> I can answer the crucial question, "Why should [name of college] admit David?" David likes the camaraderie of the basketball team who studies together and…remains abstinent during the season. I assure the Committee of Admissions that David will never use drugs, including alcohol.

This is CONFIDENTIAL, Misty. Any disclosure would haunt David when he enrolls. The spin would be that his intent was to "kiss ass" which is wrong because he did not brag. When David visited campus, he saw a member of the team who was inebriated. He notified the team captain...which takes courage....David knows the devastating impact of noxious peer pressure, but acted as he did because he knows his recovery depends on honesty. In so doing, David reinforced his sobriety. He knows that the captain of the team, who returns next year, will confront him harshly about being hypocritical if he were to relapse. Thus, he purchased insurance for his first year! Speaking of hypocrites, Misty, if the Committee of Admissions rejects David, I will take the next plane to come to campus to meet with the President and then confront your colleagues. I would be outraged if this young man were rejected because he used drugs. Only those who never used psychoactive substances possess the right to judge David's behavior.... The duration of David's drug use was brief because his parents intervened. I do not doubt, however, that had his parents been indecisive, this young man...would have escalated his use into abuse—perhaps addiction....

I would consider myself guilty of malpractice if I were to place David and/ or _____ College in a lose-lose situation. David has acquired confidence, self-respect, academic skills, and a love for learning. I believe the chances for his success exceed 95%, a statement few writers of recommendations can make.

David's growth is remarkable. The transition from destructive to constructive for this adolescent has been swift.... Momentum accelerates, motivated by wanting to purge himself of the poisonous venom of self-hatred, shame, and guilt. The basis for my optimism regarding David's recovery...is that he...knows that not only fear, frustration, and failure are ubiquitous but also how...to preserve self-respect by doing the right thing for the right reason—to maintain a proactive perspective...even when pain is pervasive by failing or being rejected.... He has the strength, knowledge, and desire to succeed.

I contend that students like David do become catalysts who can build a more nurturing and healthy environment (Bratter and Parker, 1994). Recovering students often become trusted and respected campus leaders in the dorms. Failing to persuade peers to terminate life-threatening behavior, they...will...seek help by notifying college personnel who can intervene to prevent a [crisis] before it becomes a [tragedy]. Recovering students are motivated by an awareness of the pain...they caused themselves, their families, and friends....They possess the courage to confront the destructive-dysfunctional, alienated-angry, vicious-violent behavior of classmates without worrying about being viewed by them as informers.

Recovering students can provide...security for the administration. As part of their treatment, recovering adolescents have learned the concept of responsible concern, which views intervention to be an act of friendship rather than betrayal.... They retain a vested interest to control and contain anti-social and self-destructive acts as part of their recovery. (p. 27).

The following example is excerpted from a twenty-page letter which was written to advocate why a young woman who had survived a chaotic environment should be admitted by a most competitive college.

This letter of recommendation is the most remarkable written in my career, which approaches four decades....Ilyse M.'s flaw is her SAT scores, which measure nothing more than performance on a standardized test. She received the Academic Achievement Award, given to the best student, and the History Award. She has taken the most demanding schedule in school history....Her motivation, determination, and discipline are inspiring. Ilyse states it succinctly, "I love learning!" She knows taking nine majors next term will not impress you because her grades will be submitted after, hopefully, she has been admitted.

This young woman is endowed with superior emotional and intellectual intelligence. She can succeed at whatever task(s) she thinks is/are important....Ilyse never had a chance to be normal!...Her parents divorced when she was five. Devastated by the divorce, her father related to Ilyse as if she were the adult. [There follows a detailed description of her exposure to drug use, sexual promiscuity, and emotional abuse in her mother's home, together with lack of support from other family members.]

After listening to Ilyse describe the depravity of her mother, my respect increases for this young woman. Feeling overwhelmed and lonely, she attempted suicide and became addicted to amphetamines.

I understand the intensity of her passions which motivate her to become a psychologist. What needs to be stressed, however, is Ilyse has emerged intact from toxic parents and has retained not only her innocence but also her passion to learn....

At fifteen, she had an abusive sexual relationship which ended when she had an abortion....Mrs. M. acquiesced to her daughter's demand to be emancipated by using child support checks to rent an apartment for Ilyse when she was 16. This adolescent survived economically, living by her wits. Ilyse had a relationship with a twenty-one year old. A year later, she supported herself by being a hostess who convinced patrons who were drinking in the bar to eat upstairs in the restaurant. She also worked as a sales person in a women's fine apparel store. Freed from accountability, Ilyse was narcissistic and hedonistic.

Initially, Ilyse resisted the therapeutic school. I wrote her a letter spelling out the self-destructive nature of her behavior, intending to precipitate a crisis. Rather than [leaving], Ilyse found it gratifying to help others to help themselves, at first in a detached way, but then she began to internalize her messages. Her confrontations are accurate. She possesses the intuitive genius and insight to persuade peers to change the wrongness of their ways....

Ilyse has incentive to pursue self-respect. She can identify at-risk students and knows what to do to limit self-destructiveness by confronting them and/ or notifying someone who can help. She has become a positive force....Often, her contributions in group psychotherapy qualify her to be a co-therapist! Ilyse now knows what she needs to do....I am confident she will do the right thing for the right reason(s). Her contributions to the University of _____ will be vital. Given her experience and training, she can identify potential problems before they escalate. Stated succinctly, I contend with absolute conviction Ilyse M. will be a positive, rational force who will be respected, trusted, admired, and loved by peers and professors, as has been the case at the John Dewey Academy.

I make the most emphatic assertion I have made in any letter of recommendation written....If Plato's "philosopher-king" government were in effect, and women were needed to sire children to become leaders, Ilyse M. would be [one of only three females] I would nominate. Please assure the Committee of Admissions you know that I do not exaggerate. In addition, please tell them that less than ten percent of graduates feel the need for psychotherapy or pharmacology.

I am confident Ilyse will contribute to the common good of the University of _____ by making life in the classroom and on the campus a better place....

Follow-up

If a student is rejected by one college, despite efforts to advocate for him, but excels elsewhere, I inform the office of admissions, not to gloat or verbalize bitterness, but to emphasize I have the expertise to predict success based on extensive knowledge of the applicant. This follow-up serves to foster a relationship that can benefit future applicants. Conversely, when a student fails or, worse, creates problems, I acknowledge my error. Twice, when I learned from a third party that students sold drugs on campus, I notified the president and dean of students and sent copies of the correspondence to the student and office of admissions. My purpose was not to take revenge on the student. My intent is not only to force cessation of a dangerous act but also to preserve a relationship with the college. A serendipitous payoff occurs when admissions personnel notify me about a student's problem, so I can intervene before the problem becomes a crisis or a tragedy.

Fees

Undeniably, advocacy is time consuming. In independent practice, the practitioner needs to decide in advance an equitable hourly rate or retainer structure. Families appreciate the importance of being admitted by a college of quality. Some SAT tutors charge $500 per hour. Wealthy families will contribute millions of dollars to the college to increase their child's chances to be admitted. Fees should not be contingent on admission (after all, surgeons do not charge a bonus if the patient is restored to health), nor should they be excessive. In my view, an excessive fee can prevent the formation of a positive treatment alliance because the teenager feels the therapist's only incentive is money, not genuine concern.

Transference and countertransference issues in advocacy

Countertransference is a part of psychotherapy, and being an advocate is associated with unique feelings on the part of the psychotherapist, which must be understood. Defining countertransference as "all those emotions stirred in the therapist that interfere with the conduct of the treatment," Masterson (1989b) views it as "the greatest obstacle to treatment—second only to a lack of knowledge" (p. 275). Azima (1972) asserts, "It is a myth...that any therapist can escape manifestations of countertransference reactions" (p. 244). Weiner (1975) defines countertransference as when the therapist "feels or acts toward a patient in ways that are neither part of the real relationship, rationally justified by the circumstances, nor part of the working alliance, appropriate to the terms of the treatment contract" (p. 54). If the psychotherapist tries to become a peer or feels offended that the youngster wants to wound the analyst, this signals a negative countertransference. Negative countertransference reactions may emerge when the youth frustrates, disrespects, disappoints, disobeys, and angers by acting out. Danger signs include wanting to punish the youth, feeling relief when the adolescent misses a session, and being envious of student exploits. Based on work with patients with borderline personality disorder, Adler (1985) identifies three types of countertransference that adversely affect outcome and which apply to working with alienated and angry adolescents: the therapist's "(1) wish to maintain the gratifying position of nurturing mother, (2) response to the biting attacks of the patient, and (3) wish to have a well behaved patient" (p. 148). Maltsberger and Buie (1974) advise the clinician to realize that the teenager can provoke rage and can view the advocate who enforces behavior limits as the enemy. Winnicott (1992) warns that countertransference can produce hateful feelings: "An analyst has to display all the patience and tolerance and reliability of a mother devoted to her infant, has to recognize the patient's wishes as needs, has to put aside other interests in order to be available and to be...objective, and has to seem to want to give what is really only given because of the patient's needs" (p. 48).

Perhaps the most prevalent and detrimental countertransference is the desire for gratitude and recognition for the awesome gift given to the adolescent. I deal with this directly by saying, "If you want to show your appreciation, do well; then it will be easier to convince the college to admit another. Please, send me a transcript."

A significant age differential complicates transference because often the teenager views the advocate as the parents' surrogate, who possesses the power to prevent the youth from using psychoactive substances.

As I have written:

> Most adolescents in my practice have infuriated and alienated school personnel, the clergy, employers, and agency professionals who could help them educationally and vocationally. Aggressively negotiating the most favorable deal for the adolescent is an integral part of the treatment relationship....The therapist-advocate must be prepared to assume a variety of roles: negotiator, protector, intervener, broker, supporter, representative (Bratter, 1973, p. 594).

The psychotherapist must help the adolescent resolve the symbiotic bind that he or she is in by teaching the youth self-assertive skills, thus allowing the teen to move beyond the treatment relationship. This means moving beyond the gratification provided by fantasies of the therapist's omnipotence. Adler (1985) writes:

> The omnipotence that the patient ascribes to the therapist as [the patient] recreates the mother-infant dyadic tie can give the therapist much pleasure.... As the patient works through the infantile regression and as more mature choices become open to him, he may begin to take steps away from the therapist-mother....Because...wishes cannot be totally gratified by the therapist, the patient's...rage may destroy the sense of gratification the therapist was receiving from the previous, positive relationship with the patient (1986, pp. 148–149).

The psychotherapist should avoid using advocacy to fulfill unresolved conflicts, for example, by entering into competition with parents, or wishing to punish them for neglect, or feeling that the student owes him because he has secured preferential consideration. Advocacy can become therapeutically detrimental when the psychotherapist... rob[s] the [youth] of a sense of success, of achievement, of accomplishment (Bratter, 1977).

Regardless of the therapist's theoretical orientation, his or her narcissistic needs can adversely influence outcome. When the youth remains deceitful and insulting, I respond, "I am wasting my time. I would be dishonest to deny feeling devalued and disrespected." Depending on the severity of behavior, I warn, "If your deceitful acts continue, I will consider terminating our relationship." On the one hand, the therapist needs to be cautious about issuing an ultimatum, which can create a noxious power struggle. On the other hand, however, there are consequences for irresponsible, inferior, impulsive, illicit, and dishonest acts. In extreme cases, I have rescinded recommendations, knowing this act will result in rejection of the student's application. In these cases, truth can have a compelling therapeutic and cathartic effect (Bratter, Coiner, and Parker, 2006).

The adolescent is overwhelmed by relief, joy, and pride when a college admits him or her. Never should the therapist demand appreciation or claim it is his or her victory. It does not matter whether the teenager or family express their approval. The therapist knows, which is sufficient gratification. The need for more approval makes the therapist vulnerable; this need may be traced to parental withholding of praise and approval in his or her own youth. Being on the winning team should suffice. Indulging the wish to be a hero might entice the psychotherapist to be dishonest or to exaggerate, thus endangering the brittle alliance and treatment outcome. Consumed by the guilt associated with an undeserved admission, the youth may sabotage success. Conversely, rejection by the college will provoke a negative reaction. Never blame the student for a college rejection (unless the student did not continue to progress); such criticism could prompt a premature termination of treatment.

Lessons from Shaw's *Pygmalion*

Shaw's *Pygmalion* (1916) has implications for therapists/advocates. The fictionalized professor, Henry Higgins, became involved with his student (as did Freud when he housed and fed patients). Higgins helped Eliza Doolittle improve her lot by escaping from the shackles of the lower class. Had the professor not mobilized social contacts, Eliza would have continued to sell flowers on the street.

Higgins's goal was to prove he was "the greatest teacher" (p. 40) of linguistics. He wagered Colonel Pickering he could teach Doolittle elocution and etiquette so that Eliza would be accepted as a member of the upper class. Shaw portrayed Higgins as an arrogant and egotistical bully whose primary concern was self-aggrandizement. The contemptible and irascible professor's plan was based on guile. To gratify egotistical needs, Henry reduced Eliza to an object, which prevented the formation of a helping relationship. The transference-countertransference dynamic was toxic. This negative reaction could have been avoided had Higgins felt, "I helped you to help yourself. You worked hard. You deserve the credit." Being competitive with his student, Higgins destroyed what Meeks and Bernet (1990) term "the fragile alliance." He was, however, an effective advocate, so an astute clinician can learn from the professor's errors. Eliza Doolittle's primary presenting problems were poor speech and a negative attitude that limited her professional and social options. She needed habilitation, not rehabilitation. Eliza lacked the breeding and knowledge necessary to be accepted into upper-class English society. Higgins negated Eliza's achievement by boasting that her educational and social successes were his.

Eliza: ....I've won your bet for you haven't I? That's enough for you. I don't matter.

Higgins:	You won my bet! You! Presumptuous insect! I won it!
Eliza:	What's to become of me? What's to become of me?
Higgins:	How the devil do I know?...What does it matter?
Eliza:	You don't care. You wouldn't care if I was dead. I'm nothing to you (p. 100).

Higgins earned accolades as a mentor-advocate who maintained high expectations for Eliza's improvement. But his demanding credit for Eliza's achievements crippled his effectiveness and resulted in an adversarial relationship.

The need for innovation: Not a conclusion, but a beginning

Eighty percent of students with whom I work are accepted by colleges of their first choice. Admissions personnel know I am a passionate and candid advocate. My recommendations exceed fifteen pages. I write several letters, each of which documents improvement. For the first half of my career, I was in independent practice. During the last half I have headed the John Dewey Academy, a college preparatory therapeutic boarding school, whose graduates attend competitive colleges and seventy percent graduate from these institutions of higher learning. These statistics exceed those of other schools—proof that when the advocate writes realistic and persuasive recommendations, colleges of quality will be responsive and, more importantly, recovering students can succeed.

Before a student leaves the John Dewey Academy to attend college, I write a letter with the final transcript:

> When a...self-destructive adolescent who possesses superior intellectual... potential participates in a prolonged corrective emotional experience and has returned intact from a painful detour caused by indulgent and stupid conscious choices with a positive sense of self and a need to justify his existence to himself, I am confident he will assume a positive leadership role in the classroom and on the campus. This reality justifies admission. I assert that the contributions of recovering students are more valuable than the performances of others because they frequently enhance the common good, not just that of a select few.

Recidivism is high in this treatment population because, until adolescents are convinced that diligent work can restore upward mobility, they will not invest energy to escape from self-imposed no-exit prisons in which they have entombed themselves. Unless prepared to extend treatment parameters to include advocacy, the therapist needs to decline to treat troubled and troublesome teens.

There are occupational rewards. Many adolescents achieve greatness by improving the quality of life for others. It is gratifying to know that I possess a special expertise, indefatigable resilience, and the necessary toughness to help a population of adolescents who have been viewed as untreatable and uneducable.

I love the urgency, knowing that it is the brightest and the best who reject and are rejected by an environment they feel is inimical to affective, artistic, intellectual, and moral needs. I love the therapeutic challenge of finding the symbolic key to unlock the door, and am willing to blast open the door, when indicated, by using confrontation. Only a few keys are lost. There are occupational hazards (Bratter, 2003). Four committed suicide. Four died of drug overdoses. Two were murdered for drug-related activities. I have delivered three eulogies.

Most teenagers with whom I have worked reclaim their lives from destruction and drug dependency. To paraphrase Henry Adams, a therapist can affect eternity; (s)he can never tell when his or her influence ends. It is gratifying to learn about achievements: graduation from college or graduate school, job promotions, marriage, and the birth of a child or grandchild. When attending a family celebration, it feels good to be remembered by family members and friends who comment, "You're Tom. I know you." The most important test, as my career nears its conclusion, is knowing that if I could start again, I would select the same group of adolescents with whom to work. I have few regrets. Successes significantly outnumber the failures, although this does not minimize the pain of defeat.

No research has evaluated the impact of expanding the helping relationship to include advocacy, since this is not common practice. Extending the psychotherapeutic alliance dramatically increases the probability of success when working with a population heretofore not amenable to treatment. My forty-year career supports this a priori assumption.

References

Adler, G. (1985), *Borderline Psychopathology and Its Treatment*. New York: Jason Aronson.

Aichhorn, A. (1935), *Wayward Youth*. New York: Viking Press.

Aichhorn, A. (1964), *Delinquency and Child Guidance: Selected Papers*. New York: International Universities Press.

Alexander, F. (1962), In *Science and Psychoanalysis*, ed. V. J. Masserman. New York: Grune and Stratton.

Amodeo, M. & Drouilhet (1992), Substance-abusing adolescents. In *Countertransference in Psychotherapy with Children & Adolescents*, ed. J. R. Brandell. Northvale, NJ: Jason Aronson, pp. 285–314.

Armor, D. A. & Taylor, S. E. (1998), Situated optimism: Specific outcome expectancies and self-regulation. In *Advances in Experimental Social Psychology*, ed. M. P. Zanna. New York: Academic Press, pp. 309–379.

Azima, F. (1972), Transference-countertransference issues in group psychotherapy for adolescents. *Intl. J. of Child Psychoanal.*, 1:48–57.

Blos, P. (1962), *On Adolescence: A Psychoanalytic Interpretation*. New York: Free Press of Glencoe.

Bratter, B. I., Bratter, C. J. & Bratter, T. E. (1995), Beyond reality: The need to (re)gain self-respect. *Psychother. Theory, Res. & Pract.*, 32:59–69.

Bratter, T. E. (1972), Group therapy with affluent, alienated, adolescent drug abusers. *Psychother. Theory Res. & Pract.*, 9:308–313.

Bratter, T. E. (1977), The psychotherapist as advocate: Extending the therapeutic alliance with adolescents. *J. Contemp. Psychoanal.*, 8:119–127.

Bratter, T. E. (2003), Surviving suicide: Treatment challenges working with gifted, acting-out, drug-dependent adolescents. *Intl. J. Reality Therapy,* 22:32–37.

Bratter, T. E., Bratter, C. J., Coiner, N. L., Kaufman, D. S., & Steiner, K. M. (2006), Helping gifted, defiant, and unconvinced students succeed at the John Dewey Academy. *Ethical Human: An Intl. J. of Critical Inquiry.* 8:7–16.

Bratter, T. E. & Hammerschlag, C. A. (1975), Advocate, activist, agitator: The drug abuse program administrator as a revolutionary-reformer. In *Drug Abuse Control: Administration and Politics*, ed. R. L. Rachin & E. H. Czjakoski. Lexington, MA: D. C. Heath, pp. 121–145.

Bratter, T. E. & Parker, T. H. (1994), Bright, angry, recovering students: Their gifts to colleges. *J. College Admission*, 142:23–28.

Bratter, T. E., Bratter, C. J. & Coiner, N. L. (2006) Candor, confidentiality, and the college admission of recovering students. *Internat. J. Reality Ther.*, 25:29–34.

Davis, T. & Paster, V. S. (2000), Nurturing resilience in early adolescence: A tool for future success. *J. College Student Psychol.*, 15:17–33.

Eriksen, K. (1997), *Making an Impact: A Handbook on Counselor Advocacy.* Washington, DC: Taylor & Francis.

Frankl, V. E. (1967), *Psychotherapy and Existentialism: Selected Papers on Logotherapy.* New York: Simon & Schuster.

Garmezy, N. & Rutter, M. (1983), *Stress, Coping, and Development in Children.* New York: McGraw-Hill.

Giovacchini, P. (1985), Countertransference and the severely disturbed adolescent. *Adolescent Psychiatry*, 5:449–467.

Grosser, C. F. (1965), Community development programs for serving the urban poor. *Social Work*, 17:32–39.

Hallowitz, D. (1974), Advocacy in the context of treatment. *Social Casework,* 55:416–420.

Hanna, F.J., Hanna, C. A. & Keys, S. G. (1999), Fifty strategies for counseling defiant, aggressive adolescents: Reaching, accepting, and relating. *J. Couns. & Development.*, 77:395–404.

Horney, K. (1945), *Our Inner Conflicts.* New York: W. W. Norton.

Katz, P. (1998), Establishing the therapeutic alliance. *Adolescent Psychiatry*, 23:89–105.

Luthar, S. S. & Zigler, E. (1991), Vulnerability and competence: A review of research on resilience in childhood. *Amer. J. Orthopsychiat.*, 6:6–21.

Maltsberger, J. T. & Buie, D. H. (1974), Countertransference hate in the treatment of suicidal patients. *Arch. Gen. Psychiat.*, 30:625–633.

Masterson, J. F. (1972), *Treatment of the Borderline Adolescent: A Developmental Approach.* New York: John Wiley.

Masterson, J. F. (1989a), Prologue: Evolution. In *Psychotherapy of the Disorders of the Self: The Masterson Approach*, eds. J. F. Masterson & R. Klein. New York: Brunner/Mazel, pp. xi-xx.

Masterson, J. F. (1989b), Introduction to countertransference. In *Psychotherapy of the Disorders of the Self: The Masterson Approach*, ed. J. F. Masterson & R. Klein. New York: Brunner /Mazel, pp. 275–276.

Meeks, J. E. & Bernet, W. (1990), *The Fragile Alliance: An Orientation to the Psychiatric Treatment of the Adolescent*, 4th ed. Malabar, FL: Krieger Publishing, Co.

Myers, J. E., Sweeney, T. J., & White, V. (2002). Advocacy for counseling and counselors: A professional imperative. *J. Couns. & Development*, 80:394–402.

Nagel, S. B. (1989), Addictive behavior: Problems in treatment with borderline patients. In: *Psychotherapy of the Disorders of the Self: The Masterson Approach*, eds. J. F. Masterson & R. Klein. New York: Brunner/Mazel, pp. 395–410.

Stotland, E. (1969), *Psychology of Hope: An Integration of Experimental, Clinical, & Social Approaches*. San Francisco: Jossey-Bass.

Stone, B. J. (1971), The rehabilitation counselor as client advocate. *J. Applied Rehab. Counsel.*, 2:46–54.

Taylor, M. E. Kenneny, M. E., Reed, G. M., Bower, J. E. & Greenwald, T. L. (2002), Positive resources, positive illusions, and health. *American Psychologist*, 55:99–109.

Thompson, S. C., Sobolaw-Shubin, A., Galbraith, M. E., Schwankvosky, L., & Druzen, D. (1993), Maintaining perceptions of control: Finding perceived control in low-control circumstances. *J. Personal. & Soc. Psychol.*, 64:293–304.

Vash, C. (1987), Fighting another's battles: When is it helpful? Professional? Ethical? *J. of Applied Rehabil. Counsel.*, 18:15–16.

Weiner, I. B. (1975), *Principles of Psychotherapy*. New York: John Wiley.

Williams, P. & Davis, D. (2002), *Therapist as Life Coach: Transforming Your Practice*. New York: Norton.

Winnicott, D. W. (1992), Hate in the counter-transference. In *Countertransference in Psychotherapy with Children & Adolescents*, ed. J. R. Brandell. Northvale, NJ: Jason Aronson, pp. 47–57. (Original article published 1949)

9 Confrontation—A potent psychotherapeutic approach with difficult adolescents

Thomas Edward Bratter and Lisa Sinsheimer

Abstract

This chapter describes the use of confrontation at the John Dewey Academy, a college-preparatory therapeutic boarding school. The treatment utilizes caring confrontation and positive peer pressure within a therapeutic community setting. The authors discuss the conceptual basis for the use of confrontation, drawing upon the literature about therapeutic communities. They offer a rationale for the efficacy of this psychotherapeutic approach in a population of bright adolescents who are resistant to traditional treatment. They illustrate the use of confrontation with an extended excerpt from a therapeutic group. Countertransference issues related to the use of confrontation are also discussed.

Toward a definition of clinical confrontation

Nunberg (1955) provides a reasonable definition of confrontation when he proposes the psychoanalyst "[call] the patient's attention to his inner conflicts, the sources of which are not known to either of them, and asks him to be helpful in discovering the unknown, the repressed. Thus, from the very beginning, the aims of the analyst are opposed to those of the patient, to the wishes of his repressing ego" (p. 123). Nunberg disagrees with Devereux (1951), who explicitly states that confrontation "yields no insight, and merely focuses the attention of the patient on something which he perceived but failed to register—or refuses to acknowledge openly" (p. 69).

Carkhuff and Berenson's (1967) definition has stood the test of time. They report that confrontation helps the person understand:

> himself, his strengths and resources, as well as his self-destructive behavior....It is a challenge to... become integrated....It is directed at discrepancies... between what the client says and does...and between illusion and reality....It implies a constructive attack upon an unhealthy confederation of miscellaneous illusions, fantasies, and life avoidance techniques in order to create a reintegration at a higher level of health (p. 171).

Confrontation in self-help therapeutic communities

During World War II at Henderson Hospital in the Belmont Social Rehabilitation Unit in England, Rapoport (1960), a sociologist, was the first to describe group psychotherapy to be "reality confrontation." Shankman (1978) provides a description of the self-help therapeutic community (TC), as illustrated by Casriel (1963); Bratter (1978); Bratter, Collabolletta, Fossbender, Pennacchia, and Rubel (1985); Glaser (1974); Sugarman (1974, 1986); and Yablonsky (1965), in which recovered persons act as catalysts and responsible role models:

> The TC might best be described as a school which educates people who have never learned how to live or feel worthy without hurting themselves and others. The therapeutic community helps people who have tried again and again to get what they wanted from life and have continually defeated themselves. The principle combines the basic and universal human values of knowledge, love, honesty, and work, with the dynamic instrument of intense group pressure, in order to recognize and help correct personality defects which prevent people from living by these values. The results lie in rehabilitation so that the individual may reenter his or her community as an independent and productive person (p. 156).

When describing self-help peer psychotherapy, Van Stone and Gilbert (1972) candidly describe the brutality of confrontation in residential therapeutic communities that are run by recovering addicts. Confrontations needed to be harsher in these adult communities than they would be with teenagers, and justifiably so:

> [Confrontation is] a kind of group therapy in which each member is...presented with candid, personal facts regarding every observable behavior or attitude recognized by the group as being self-defeating or dishonest. If the member...attempts to explain or deny any observation, he is ridiculed...and insulted as his fellow members hammer away at the distorted ideas that he offers in support of his damaging behavior patterns. Intellectual insight or genetic self-interpretations are derided as an escape from responsibility for current behavior. Honesty, trust in the group, realistic self-assessment, appropriate emotional release, and changed behavior, in particular, are rewarded by sympathetic counsel and encouragement from fellow members (p. 585).

The professional community initially characterized confrontation as cruel. Maslow (1967), the progenitor of humanistic psychology, recognized the effectiveness of confrontation after attending groups at Synanon, the first ex-addict-administered therapeutic community. He wrote, "people are ...tough.... They can take a...lot....I've suggested that a name for this might be 'no crap therapy.' It...clean[s] out defenses [and] rationalizations." (p. 28). Ruitenbeek (1970) agrees with Maslow, describing the essence of this technique as an "insistence upon total honesty....No rationalizations...are allowed" (p. 166). The clinical challenge of confrontation is to help the youth commit to accept responsibility by converting noxious emotions into constructive acts via the internalization of positive values. Self-respect and success become positive addictions.

Confrontation is painful because it penetrates protective barriers. Using a psychoanalytic orientation, Adler (1985) defines confrontation as an attempt to "gain a patient's attention to inner experiences or perceptions of outer reality of which he is conscious or is about to be made conscious" (p. 122). Sifneos (1991) cautions that the therapist who uses confrontation needs to:

> "be convinced that the patient is able to withstand [much] stress....[Effective] confrontation must be based on the therapist's observation about a series of paradoxical behavioral patterns, contradictory statements....It must motivate him to look at himself from a different point of view" (pp. 374, 382). Cohen (1982), who reconciles confrontation and psychoanalysis, provides a comprehensive synthesis when he contends that "confrontation analysis is a method of investigating, analyzing, and evaluating human behavior in the context of interpersonal interaction. It...contains a theoretical framework within which to understand the evolution, maintenance, and modifications of personality dimensions" (p. xv).

Countertransference issues

Collabolletta, Gordon, and Kaufman (1998) stress that the therapist's intent determines whether the confrontation is therapeutic or an abuse of power: "When the psychotherapist's intent is to promote change, this kind of confrontation becomes caring and constructive." When the intent is to prevent a student from engaging in destructive, dangerous, and deceitful acts, compassionate confrontation becomes the most potent expression of responsible concern. A skillful confrontation provides prima facie proof of the therapist's care and emotional investment.

The therapist needs to be mindful of potential countertransferential contamination when using this technique. Only the confronter knows personal motivations; thus, one must understand the psychodynamics before confronting. Unresolved countertransferential issues can provoke cruel confrontations. Giovacchini (1985) notes that adolescents can arouse disruptive countertransference reactions because of the intensity of their neediness and defiance, and warns that countertransference may destroy the treatment relationship, or it may lead to therapeutically beneficial insights. The therapist can feel jealous that these adolescents have emancipated themselves from middle-class restraints. Or, more likely, be disgusted by cruel and feel a need to punish the offender. Consultation with colleagues or a supervisor can minimize the likelihood of acting out a destructive countertransference reaction.

Sequence and principles of confrontation

Bratter (2003) asserts that "there are two sequential phases to confrontation: first, the unlearning of dysfunctional attitudes and acts and, second, learning healthy responses. Confrontation can penetrate the permissive and indulgent attitudes of families that [created] the psychopathology of alienation, deceit, irresponsibility, and self-absorbed behaviors" (p. 140).

Bratter (1977, p. 170) lists seven principles of confrontation psychotherapy:

1. Attack the malignant and dysfunctional aspects of behavior.
2. Penetrate the facade of justification of behavior.
3. Force individuals to accept responsibility for behavior.
4. Help persons evaluate their behavior.
5. Assist individuals to be aware and to anticipate the consequences and pay-offs of their behavior.
6. Challenge persons to mobilize their resources.
7. Define a direction so that persons can continue their growth and development.

How confrontation facilitates change in adolescents

Confrontation is a potent psychotherapeutic process designed to help the adolescent not only to recognize (and change) the self-destructive aspects of behavior but also to acquire skills that help actualize potential. In a group setting, peers offer insight and suggestions, thus providing the catalytic conditions necessary for self-exploration and improvement. Confrontation pierces the formidable protective armor of denial, deceit, and distortion. Meeks and Bernet (1990) note "accurate confrontation is much easier in the inpatient setting than it is in the treatment of outpatient adolescents" (p. 578). Johnson (1985) views confrontation as supplying an "observing ego" (p. 255). Brook (1996) believes that confrontation helps adolescent "group members...to confront denial and accept responsibility for their actions" (p. 258).

Bratter (1972) describes the therapeutic thrust of a confrontation-group orientation:

> Using a confrontation-teaching-interpretative-reasoning approach, the group demonstrates to the [member] the irresponsible and self-defeating aspects of...behavior [and]...begins to understand the consequences of his acts and attempts to become more responsible to himself, others, and society. Emphasis is placed on the *eigenwelt* (the relation to one's self)—i.e., the immediate experience. The individual must acknowledge his perceptions of the conflict, the problem, his irresponsibility, etc....

The individual, gaining the candid opinions and admonishments of his peers regarding the more destructive elements of his behavior, considers a new orientation and behavior (p. 309).

Confrontation can:

- Expedite a behavioral change—i.e., stop dangerous and dysfunctional behavior.
- "Force" the adolescent to be accountable for attitudes and acts.
- Help students understand future consequences and payoffs for current behavior.
- Mobilize personal talents to actualize potential.

Confrontation utilizes provocative questions to stimulate self evaluation. Do your attitudes and acts help you to achieve your intermediate and long-term goals? How do others view you? Do you have self-respect? In addition, the therapist must elicit reactions from the confronted and group members about their reactions to the confrontation. Garner (1970) urges the therapist to ask frequently, "What do you think or feel about what I told you?" (p. 231).

Helping each other while helping the self

To minimize the impact of negative countertransference reactions, since a significant age differential exists between adolescents and the group leader, peers are encouraged to do most of the confronting. Volkman and Cressey (1963), among the first to recognize the importance of self-help confrontational psychotherapy groups, write:

> The most effective mechanism for exerting group pressure on members will be found in groups so organized that criminals are induced to join with non-criminals for the purpose of changing other criminals. A group in which criminal "A" joins with some non-criminals to change criminal "B" is probably more effective in changing criminal "A" (p. 139).

Brager (1965) notes increased self esteem in group members when they confront peers to better themselves. Reisman (1965) labels this treatment dynamic as "the helper principle," and notes that the helper often gains more from the helping process than the person being helped. Positive peer pressure traces its antecedents to self-help psychotherapy. Hurvitz (1970) reports that when peers are active,

> they focus on the presenting problem, and assume that by following principles and methods of their movement, they will help each member solve his specific problem....They may ridicule and attack each other with great hostility and they may provoke aggressive and hostile feelings; however, peers

regard such attacks and provocations as other's expressions of concern and concern (p. 44).

Use of confrontation at the John Dewey Academy

Bratter, Sinsheimer, and Kaufman, in chapter 7 of this volume, have described the population and treatment philosophy at the John Dewey Academy (JDA). As they have said, JDA youth are "immune to traditional therapeutic and teaching techniques. They have erected formidable barriers and defenses which need to be cracked before they will think rationally....Peers confront each other by demanding that each member accept accountability for immature, irresponsible, illicit, and self-destructive acts" (p. 73).

Compassionate confrontation: Rebutting the critics

When entering the John Dewey Academy, most students possess toxic attitudes that reduce others to objects to satisfy voracious narcissistic needs, self-entitlement, and self- aggrandizement. Both traditional therapeutic approaches and the administration of psychotropic medicine have proven ineffective. No chemical imbalance exists. Many Dewey youth have a virulent attitude that renders psychotherapy ineffective which explains why recidivism rates are high.

Critics contend that confrontation is controversial, counter therapeutic, and cruel punishment which often brutalizes persons-in-treatment. Confrontation attempts to modify irresponsible, impulsive, immature, stupid and self-destructive behavior. Confrontation penetrates denial, distortion, and dysfunctional attitudes. Critics protest, furthermore, that the use of confrontation is prompted by a negative countertransference reaction. Confrontation has been labeled "attack therapy" for pejorative reasons. Opponents of "attack therapy" do not understand is that confrontation has proven effective to eradicate malignant, dangerous, vicious attitudes and acts. While some critics condemn confrontation to be "cruel," they need to remember that Dewey students have engaged in dangerous, often death-defying behavior which demands heroic intervention. Unless the therapist can persuade the youth to avoid a collision course with disaster, there can be profoundly serious consequences. The primary goal of psychotherapy is to preserve life, so desperate and heroic treatment interventions are required for this difficult-to-treat population. When viewed from this humanistic perspective, confrontation connotes caring by the therapist who attempts to convince the adolescent to become more responsible, responsive, and respectful.

Similar to other medical procedures, there are abuses of confrontation psychotherapy which the authors acknowledge and condemn. The authors, therefore, do not minimize the noxious impact of confrontation when done for the wrong reasons.

There are similarities between the psychotherapist who confronts, the radiologist who medicates, the surgeon who operates, and the psychiatrist who prescribes psychotropic medication. Stated simply, these procedures are subject to abuse. In addition, each procedure attempts to attack malignancies. If the truth be known, confrontation is more benign than other medical approaches. The surgeon, radiologist, and psychiatrist do more physical and permanent damage under the guise of medical treatment than does the therapist who confronts. Interesting, these professions escape criticism because the end is thought to justify the means. There are more malpractice suits against medical professionals than psychotherapists who confront.

Confrontation psychotherapy: A case study

As an illustration, we present an excerpt of our group process. Prior to attending JDA, Jason had been diagnosed as having schizoaffective disorder and had been prescribed a cocktail of psychotropic medications, including amphetamines, antidepressants, and anxiolytics. Jason's father died when he was twelve, and his mother was in remission from a brain tumor. He witnessed several people jumping to their deaths from the World Trade Center towers during the 9/11 terror attacks. Two years ago, Jason learned he had the same hereditary cardiac condition that caused his father's premature death, and he underwent the implantation of a pacemaker-defibrillator.

Considering his history, post-traumatic stress disorder might have been a more appropriate diagnosis. Regardless of diagnosis, however, this boy had clear explanations for his choice to suppress his feelings and for his decision not to trust others. He struggled with a continuing sense of abandonment and betrayal, stemming from his father's sudden death. During the 18 months that he was at JDA, he remained closed off from other students and staff. The following is a fragment of a group session in which first the group leader and then the other members of the group confronted Jason on his behavior and their reactions to it. Before convening this group and implementing this confrontation, the group leader discussed the treatment impasse extensively with colleagues. The intent of this confrontation was to precipitate a crisis, forcing Jason to change or to leave.

Leader: Jason, recently adults have asked if I think you are organically damaged since you refuse to heed repeated warnings not only to change but also to become a contributing member of the community. I admit that for the first time I mentioned that perhaps they are right and I am wrong. Maybe you *are* damaged goods and are incapable of changing. You might be the first student in our twenty-year history who needs medication to function. I intend to recommend to your mother that you be evaluated by a psychiatrist who specializes in pharmacology.

Jason: I am not. You know damn well I'm not crazy and don't need that crap.

Leader: I no longer know what to think. What I do know is that you have been here for eighteen months, but haven't changed much. You still isolate.

	You still refuse to relate. You still don't trust anyone. You still are stubborn. But to your credit, you finally have started to do well academically. I think you hide in your academics by claiming you need to study six or seven hours a day.
Jason:	Yes, but…
Leader:	Yes period. Your classmates complain that you're a drag and a drain. They don't want to waste their time and energy reaching out to you and having you reject them. Ask them.
Jason:	I've been talking to people. (He lists five students.)
Mary:	Big deal. They are new students. None have been here longer than three months. What about us? We know you much better than they do. They don't know how to confront you. So you continue to play stupid games.
Laurie:	I have no idea who you are. When you feel uncomfortable and threatened, you shut down. When my father died abruptly from a heart attack, just like your father, you never even said you were sorry. This is why I stopped pursuing you.
Jason:	I don't want to talk to you because you don't want to talk to me.
Leader:	That's a very mature response. You're right, but do you know why?
Jason:	No.
Leader:	You lie. You know damn well. Everyone is frustrated and weary. They have extended themselves by sharing experiences and confronting you. What have they gotten from you? Only silence and sarcasm. So they finally said to themselves, 'Fuck him. He's simply not worth it.' You quit. No, that's wrong. You never tried.
Allie:	Tom's right. I quit six months ago. I gave you the benefit of the doubt that, underneath your defenses, you were caring. I don't believe that any more. You talk in a monotone. I cannot remember when I felt you cared. You are the most frightened and self-absorbed person I've ever met. I know why. When I came I was too scared to care. I had a damn good excuse. I had several abusive relationships with guys. I felt sorry for myself and saw myself as the victim. I was confronted that it was my choice. I chose to remain with these abusive jerks when I should have rejected them! It was scary to trust because I feared the worst. Yeah, I got hurt once or twice. I was knocked down. But I got up and tried again. And you know what? Today, I have the best friends I ever had.
Laurie:	I don't blame Allie for not giving a damn. No one trusts you. You are nineteen. You continue to treat your mother like she's the enemy! You abuse your younger sister. None of us care whether you leave or stay. I pity you. You are too scared to be human. You are a poor excuse for a person.
Eddie:	Jason, it's really that easy. You lack the guts to venture forth. You're a coward. I'd lie if I said I care because I don't. Blame yourself. But what

frightens me is that I know if you don't do it at JDA, you never will. You will never be in an environment which is so caring and safe.

Paul: Eddie's understating your problem. Several of us believe you have major guilt, but lack the integrity to take accountability. Fuck your fears. Take accountability. Things can't get much worse.

Shirley: Do you know what I think the problem is?

Leader: No. Tell us.

Shirley: Jason does not believe you will expel him. You've threatened so many times to expel him that he thinks he's immune.

Eddie: Shirley's right. Jason knows you like bright students, so he's gambling since he has not done anything expellable, you'll let him graduate.

Leader: Jason, if this is what you think, your reality testing is flawed. Complete the next two weeks and then go home for the holidays. Think about what you will want to do with your life. And then write a ten-page essay why I should readmit you. Include in this document your guilt and what you will change.

Allie: Why wait? He thinks you are bluffing. He's not going to change. For the next two weeks, he will do nothing.

Leader: You're right, Allie. Jason, leave in three days. I will give you seventy-two hours to make arrangements because I doubt your mother will permit you to return home. My guess is that all the New York City homeless shelters are filled because it's cold, but I suggest you call them.

Paul: We're wasting our time. We have confronted you many times but you ignored us. You have made commitments to change, but you never have. You continue to joke and act nonchalant. You've done this for six months, so I agree with what Tom said at the beginning of the group. Maybe you just don't get it! I believe you lack the guts to come out from behind all the barriers you have erected. You will be a lonely guy who becomes bitter because no one will be knocking at the door asking you to let us in. Maybe you should watch Dickens' "Christmas Carol." You could become Scrooge.

Susan: I've kept quiet because I tried many times to reach out to you, but you always gave me shit. You continue to be obnoxious and confront others about dumb shit which tells everyone to stay away. I know when I confront kids rather than connecting with them, they get the message to stay away.

Leader: Sadly, I doubt if this group will have much impact. You have heard all this shit many, many times. This may be the last group you attend at John Dewey. I won't shed any tears if you do not return, other than we failed to help you in your time of desperate need. But Scrooge changed when he was much older than you are. Unfortunately, Scrooge is a fictional character. Maybe you ought to read Dickens when you go home. Unless you change by letting the sun shine in, you very well could become Scrooge. It would be tragic if you were to live a wasted life because you have been blessed with awesome intelligence. You could have been great. You could have improved the quality of life. But you won't unless you get the guts to show you care. It's late, but there still is time. The next month will be the most important in your life, because the decisions you make will influence you until you die. I hope for your sake, and that of society, you finally make the right decisions because this may be your last chance. Enough. I don't want to waste any more time. I end abruptly because I do not want to have closure. I hope you are scared because I am scared for you! You can win, but time is a precious commodity, which you lack.

Case follow-up

Following this group, Jason enrolled in a four-week wilderness program in an attempt to earn readmission to Dewey. During his stay at the wilderness program, Jason received notification of early-decision admission to a prestigious college of engineering, as well as word that he had been awarded a substantial scholarship.

While in the wilderness program, Jason was admitted early decision to a prestigious engineering college. We thought this would provide the incentive for him not only to return to John Dewey but also to confront his fears. However, when he returned from the wilderness program, Jason remained intransigent. He engaged in provocative behavior, which forced his expulsion for safety reasons. He "played" with the fire alarm. He "played" with the stove, turning it on and off. He asked the dean of students if he could set fires by using his bow and drill, a skill he had learned in the wilderness. His intent seemed obvious—rather than leaving school voluntarily, Jason wanted to be expelled. It seemed certain that the behavior would escalate if he were allowed to remain. The decision to expel Jason was in keeping with the treatment principle that there are consequences for behavior. Students, parents, and staff were notified before any action was taken, and no one disagreed with the decision to expel him.

The president was faced with the dilemma of whether, and how, to report Jason's behavior to the engineering college. One option would have been to hide behind the shield of confidentiality, but it was felt that unsafe behavior does not warrant confidentiality. Additionally, notification was justified because Jason dropped four courses, which, if not explained, would have resulted in his acceptance being rescinded. Finally, there was the importance of maintaining a relationship with this college so others could attend.

At the same time, the president was aware of his reactions to Jason, which included disappointment, betrayal, anger at not being appreciated for convincing the college to grant a generous scholarship, and rage at being placed in a most uncomfortable position. He knew no one would criticize him if he urged the college to rescind admission, but knew this consequence was extreme since the family could not afford to pay tuition. It is dubious if Jason would have attended college. After careful consideration, the president wrote a letter to the dean of admissions at the college, explaining the reasons for the expulsion, reviewing the factors in Jason's background that have made it difficult for him to succeed academically and socially, and recommending that he reapply to JDA and complete a postgraduate year before attempting college. Included in the letter were the following statements.

> Please be advised...if I thought Jason were "too dangerous" or "too sick," not only would I notify _____ college, but also would refuse to give him the option to return to Dewey....Jason's refusal to comply is motivated by fear to trust others and to be emotionally vulnerable, not defiance. The only time Jason cried was when he was confronted about his reluctance to trust...because he feared friends would abandon and betray him....If permitted to attend college, I suggest Jason be required to continue psychotherapy. He needs to resolve his fear of intimacy, not because he is a threat to safety. Jason and his mother will receive a copy of this letter, so hopefully both will communicate with you. I warned Jason that [college] may rescind his acceptance....
>
> I would be willing to accompany Jason for a conference, with anyone you think makes sense, to discuss options. Undeniably, Jason is a disappointment, but I hasten to mention that several have graduated in Jason's position needing to do more work therapeutically. In college, they excelled. His prognosis remains guarded....I conclude...by stating that he has learned much.

The president would have been wrong to suggest rejection essentially because the decision is that of the college, not the preparatory school. To recommend rejection would have been an abuse of psychotherapeutic power. Post hoc, the president knew that had he become retaliatory, his motivation would have been revenge for Jason's disrespect and lack of appreciation regarding his advocacy, which had resulted in Jason's being awarded a $160,000 four-year scholarship. Had he urged that Jason be rejected, which was warranted, Jason's future would have been ruined, because without a scholarship, it would have been impossible for him to attend college. The president retained his therapeutic integrity by reporting what happened, but refraining from recommending any action. The college decided to continue to extend its offer of admission and a scholarship, and Jason plans to completed the required work and attended. Subsequently, he attained a 3.8 average which puts him on the dean's list. The president assumed an aggressive advocate stance, advocating that he become a resident assistant in the dorms. Jason has visited the John Dewey Academy six times during the year because he wants to "give back" to the school which helped him mature. He has forgiven the president and now recognizes the confrontations were expressions of concern.

Discussion

It is premature to know whether Jason will be a "success" or a "failure." Undeniably, Jason was helped by confrontation because he excelled and was admitted by a college of quality. How much has this adolescent grown, and what the quality of his interpersonal relationships will be, has not been determined. Judicious handling of this complicated situation has avoided the preclusion of future educational, professional, and social successes.

This kind of confrontation is justified when the adolescent remains intransigent or engages in extremely dangerous behavior. Alexander (1950) describes a patient who was irritating and engaged in regressive behavior. When the patient complained that no one liked him, rather than commiserating, Alexander opines that no one liked him because he was unpleasant. Subsequently the patient established a positive treatment alliance. Hearing the truth from a caring professional enabled the patient to trust and to move forward. Corwin (1991) labels this kind of intervention heroic: "When such statement is made, it is an emergency situation....The analyst knows it, the patient is...aware....But both know the moment it is uttered that it may have a prophetic significance for the patient....It implies that a psychic reaction must lead toward the establishment of a working alliance" (p. 83). We have utilized this sort of radical intervention for six seniors in past years, all of whom eventually returned to graduate. We believe Jason will not be an exception.

Critics contend that confrontation is controversial, counter therapeutic, and cruel punishment which often brutalizes persons-in-treatment. Confrontation attempts to modify irresponsible, impulsive, immature, stupid and self-destructive behavior. Confrontation penetrates denial, distortion, and dysfunctional attitudes. Critics protest, furthermore, that the use of confrontation is prompted by a negative countertransference reaction. Confrontation has been labeled "attack therapy" for pejorative reasons. Opponents of "attack therapy" do not under-stand is that confrontation has proven effective to eradicate malignant, dangerous, vicious attitudes and acts. While some critics condemn confrontation to be "cruel," they need to remember that Dewey students have engaged in dangerous, often death-defying behavior which demands heroic intervention. Unless the therapist can persuade the youth to avoid a collision course with disaster, there can be profoundly serious consequences. The primary goal of psychotherapy is to preserve life, so desperate and heroic treatment interventions are required for this difficult-to-treat population. When viewed from this humanistic perspective, confrontation connotes caring by the therapist who attempts to convince the adolescent to become more responsible, responsive, and respectful.

Conclusion

We have described a confrontation as a key aspect of a non-medically oriented residential therapeutic community. In our view, confrontation in the context of residential treatment is a potent psychotherapeutic tool that produces not only the acquisition of prosocial values but also behavioral improvement. Since these changes are internalized, long-term prognosis is quite good. Although we have no long-term systematic follow-up, anecdotal data confirm a less-than-ten-percent recidivism rate, which, to the best of our knowledge, is unmatched at any other residential treatment program. Bratter et al. (2006) contend "critics claim that confrontation psychotherapy is painful and simplistic. But they cannot explain how and why adolescents, who were extreme casualties, improve in a confrontational treatment milieu with escalating expectations for intellectual excellence and moral integrity [that] can be achieved without compromising one for the other" (p. 14). Confrontation as a psychotherapeutic technique has a long history in self-help therapeutic communities. In our experience, it can also be very effective in promoting change in adolescents who are resistant to other treatment approaches. Clearly, confrontation warrants further study.

References

Adler, G. (1985), *Borderline Psychopathology and Its Treatment*. New York: Jason Aronson.

Alexander, F. & French, T. (1946), *Psychoanalytic Therapy*. New York: Ronald Press.

Brager, G., (1965), The indigenous worker: A new approach to the social work technician. *Social Work*, 10: 33–40.

Bratter, T. E. (1972), Confrontation group psychotherapy with affluent, alienated drug abusing adolescents. *Psychother.: Theory, Res. & Pract.*, 9: 308–313.

Bratter, T. E. (1977), Confrontation groups: The therapeutic community's gift to psychotherapy. In *Proceedings of the First World Conference on Therapeutic Communities*, ed. P. Vamos & J. J. Devlin. Montreal, Canada: Portage Press, pp. 164–174.

Bratter, T. E. (1978), The four 'Rs' of the American self-help therapeutic community: Rebirth, responsibility, reality and respect. In *Proceedings of the Third World Conference on Therapeutic Communities*, ed. J. Corelli, I. Bonfiglio, T. Pediconi, & M. Collumb. Rome: International Council of Alcoholism and Addictions Press, pp. 434–448.

Bratter, T. E., Collabolletta, E., Fossbender, A. J., Pennacchia, M. C, & Rubel, J. R. (1985), The American self-help residential therapeutic community: A pragmatic treatment approach for addicted character-disordered individuals. In *Alcoholism and Substance Abuse: Strategies for Clinical Intervention*, ed. T. E. Bratter & G. G. Forrest. New York: Free Press, pp. 461–507.

Bratter, T. E. (2003), Group psychotherapy with gifted, self-destructive, drug-dependent, unconvinced adolescents. *Group*, 27: 131–146.

Bratter, T. E., Bratter, C. J., Coiner, N. L., & Steiner, K. M. (2006), Motivating gifted, defiant, and unconvinced students to succeed at the John Dewey Academy. *Ethical Human Psychology and Psychiatry*, 8: 7–16.

Brook, W. (1996), Adolescents who abuse substances. In *Group Therapy with Adolescents*, ed. P. Kymissis & D. A. Halpern. Washington, DC: American Psychiatric Association, pp. 243–264.

Carkhuff, R. R. & Berenson, R. G. (1967), *Beyond Counseling and Therapy*. New York: Holt, Rinehart and Winston.

Casriel, D. (1963), *So Fair a House: The Story of Synanon*. Englewood Cliffs, NJ: Prentice-Hall.

Cohen, A. I., (1982), *Confrontation Analysis: Theory and Practice*. New York: Grune & Stratton.

Corwin, H. A. (1991), Therapeutic confrontation from routine to heroic. In *Confrontation in Psychotherapy*, eds. G. Adler & P. G. Myerson. Northvale, NJ: Jason Aronson. pp. 69–94.

Devereux, G. (1951), Some criteria for the timing of confrontations and interpretations. *Intl. J. Psychoanal.*, 32:19–24.

Gans, J. S. & Weber, R. L. (2000), The detection of shame in group psychotherapy: Uncovering the hidden emotion. *Intl. J. Group Psychother.*, 50:381–396.

Garner, H. H. (1970), *Psychotherapy: Confrontation Problem-Solving Technique.* St Louis: Warren H. Green.

Glaser, F. B. (1974), Some historical and theoretical background of a self-help addiction treatment program. *Amer. J. Drug & Alcohol Abuse*, 1:37–52.

Giovacchini, P. (1985), Countertransference and the severely disturbed adolescent. *Adolescent Psychiatry*, 12:449–467.

Hurvitz, N. (1970), Peer self-help groups and their implications for psychotherapy. *Psychother. Theory, Prac. Res.*, 7:41–47.

Johnson, S. M. (1985), *Characterological Transformation: The Hard Work Miracle.* New York: Norton.

Kaufman, G. (1989), *The Psychology of Shame: Theory and Treatment of Shame-Based Syndromes.* New York: Springer.

Maslow, A. H. (1967), Synanon and eupsychia. *J. Humanistic Psychol.*, VII:21–32.

Meeks, J. E. & Bernet, W. (1990), *The Fragile Alliance: An Orientation to the Psychiatric Treatment of the Adolescent.* Malabar, FL: Krieger Publishing.

Nunberg, H. (1955), *Principles of Psychoanalysis.* New York: International Universities.

Reisman, F. (1965), The "helper" therapy principle. *Social Work*, 10:27–32.

Ruitenbeek, H. (1970), *The New Group Therapies.* New York: Avon Books.

Shankman, S. (1978), Criteria and factors affecting admission into and completion of the therapeutic community program. In *Proceedings of the Third World Conference on Therapeutic Communities*, ed. J. Corelli, T. Bonfiglio, T. Pediconi, & M. Collumb. Rome: Centro Italiano di Solidarieta, pp. 156–160.

Sugarman, B. (1974), *Daytop Village: A Therapeutic Community.* New York: Holt, Rinehart, and Winston.

Sugarman, B. (1986), Structure, variations, and context: A sociological view of the therapeutic community. In *Therapeutic Communities for Addictions: Readings in Theory, Research and Practice*, ed. G. De Leon & J. T. Ziegenfuss. Springfield, IL: Charles C. Thomas, pp. 65–82.

Van Stone, W. W. & Gilbert, R. (1972), Peer confrontation groups: What, why, and whether. *Amer. J. Psychiat.*, 129:581–591.

Volkman, R. & Cressey, D. R., (1963), Differential association and the rehabilitation of drug addicts. *Amer. J. Soc.*, 69:131–141.

Yablonsky, L. (1965), *The Tunnel Back: Synanon.* New York: Macmillan.

10 What's old is new
Motivational interviewing for adolescents

Lois T. Flaherty

Abstract

Motivational interviewing, developed in the substance abuse field as an approach to alcohol use, has been extended to other kinds of substance abuse and other disorders that have an addictive quality. It is a brief intervention that can be incorporated into a single session and used in non-psychiatric settings. In recent years it has been widely used for adolescents in a variety of venues, with promising results.

Introduction

Two groups of alcoholics received either one counseling session or several months of in- and outpatient treatment. One year later there were no significant differences in outcome between the two groups.

Edwards et al., 1977, p. 1004

Foremost in my mind is how it works at all....How could it possibly be, then, that a session or two of asking clients to verbalize their own suffering and reasons for change would unstuck a behavior pattern that has been so persistent.

Miller, 1996, p. 840

Motivational interviewing (MI) involves five basic techniques: (1) open-ended, (2) reflective listening, (3) eliciting self-motivational statements, (4) supportive and affirming statements, and (5) summary statements. (See Appendix 10.A.)

According to its developer, William Miller, (MI) was discovered by accident. He found, when studying an intervention for problem drinkers in the 1970s, that control groups did as well as treatment groups. In the process of unraveling what was going on in the control groups that received an initial assessment, encouragement, and advice, he was able to tease out what seemed to be the ingredients that resulted in changing their behavior. Not all of the controls improved, but those who did had counselors who were empathetic and non-confrontational, and who gave helpful information. The kind of information that seemed to be most useful was the creating of a discrepancy between the client's stated goals and his current behavior. There was no urging of the client to make changes, but rather an emphasis that the decision about whether to change was up to the client, and that he could do so whenever he was ready.

From that beginning, MI was developed into protocols and tested in a variety of situations. Books and journal articles appeared, although it remained largely unknown outside of psychiatric literature. Perhaps it was deemed too simple, or perhaps because it was developed in the addictions field, which has historically developed independently of psychiatry, it did not make it into the mainstream. But a brief intervention that appeared to work for a variety of problems with diverse patients and required little formal training was bound to spread. In a 1990 report, the Institute of Medicine recommended brief intervention, namely MI, for all patients with alcohol problems (Institute of Medicine, 1990).

A therapeutic approach that respected patients' autonomy and decision-making capacity, and was encouraging and supportive, while at the same time providing feedback about the person's current situation with respect to where she wants to be eventually, would appear to be a natural fit for adolescents. This, in fact, proved to be the case. Between 2000 and 2005, 38 articles on MI with adolescents in various contexts appeared in English language peer-reviewed journals indexed in PubMed®. The reported settings range from adolescent inpatient units to Internet chat rooms (Institute of Medicine, 1990; Woodruff, Edwards, Conway, & Elliott, 2001). While most of these articles describe pilot studies, their number indicates a growing popularity of MI in a variety of psychiatric and non-psychiatric situations.

Conditions in which MI has been studied

MI was originally developed to treat alcohol use disorders, and has been extensively studied in this context, first in adults (Edwards et al., 1977) and more recently in adolescents (Baer, Kivlahan, Blume, McKnight, & Marlatt, 2001; Bailey, Baker, Webster, & Lewin, 2004; Boekeloo et al., 2004; Collins, Carey, and Sliwinski, 2002; Gregor et al., 2003; Hungerford et al., 2003; Kelly, Donovan, Chung, Cook, & Delbridge, 2004; Larimer et al., 2001; and Stewart et al., 2005). MI has been used for marijuana use and dependence (Edwards et al., 1977) as well as for addictions to heroin and other drugs (Battjes et al., 2004; Breslin, Li, Sdao-Jarvie, Tupker, & Ittig-Deland, 2002; Kavanagh et al., 2004; Levy, Vaughan, & Knight, 2002; Spoth, Redmond, and Shin, 2001; Tait & Hulse, 2003; Tait and Hulse, 2005; Tevyaw & Monti, 2004). Extension of the early work on substance abuse led to trials of MI with other kinds of behavior that are viewed as having an addictive or habitual component, including smoking (Brown et al., 2003) and obesity (Kirk, Scott, and Daniels, 2005). Other situations not characterized by compulsive behavior in which MI has been tested are adherence to antiretroviral treatment (DiIorio, Resnicow, McDonnell et al., 2003), dietary adherence (Berg-Smith, Stevens, Brown et al., 1999), diabetes and other long term medical care (Channon, Smith, and Gregory, 2003; Aliotta, Vlasnik, and Delor, 2004), and avoidance of dental care in older adolescents, evidently a significant problem (Skaret, Weinstein, Kvale et al., 2003).

What do we know about MI?

Miller observed that a confrontational stance on the part of the therapist increased the client's resistance. Challenging the patient's assertions, disbelieving, criticizing, or arguing were all counterproductive, decreasing the likelihood that a patient would want to change. These observations led him to reframe "resistance" and "denial" as arising from interpersonal interactions, rather than qualities that resided inherently in patients. His reframing led to a conceptualization of motivation also as a dynamic interpersonal process resulting from the relationship.

Miller noted that, in contrast to the negative, resistance-increasing actions on the part of ineffective therapists, successful therapists behaved in an empathetic, supportive way, engaging in reflective listening and offering positive feedback. For example, they offered advice about community resources and discussed ways to change. They monitored readiness to change and did not push clients to change before they were ready. In psychological parlance, they enhanced self-efficacy and elicited motivational statements from their clients. Finally, they fostered an awareness of the difference between current reality and the person's own stated goals for him- or herself. This awareness of difference, termed cognitive dissonance, has been suggested as the crucial active ingredient in motivational interviewing (Draycott and Dubbs, 1998). In sum, what the therapists provided was a combination of modes of interaction (the supportive, nonjudgmental stance) and techniques (the advice and creation of cognitive dissonance).

The transtheoretical model of change

MI is closely tied to the transtheoretical model of change (TMC) which was, in fact, developed simultaneously with MI by Prochaska and DiClemente (1982). TMC was based on their review of many types of therapy and their empirical observations of smokers who were able to stop by themselves (see Rosner, 2005, for a more complete discussion of TMC). The idea here is that it is possible to categorize stages in the process by which individuals (and even institutions) undergo change. These stages apply to all change and occur regardless of what method or theory is invoked to explain the change. MI can be used at any stage, but its appropriate use depends on an awareness of at what level of change a person is.

Moderators of MI

Prior conditions have an effect on the outcome of MI. These include pretreatment substance abuse history, school adjustment, and emotional abuse history. Lack of prior treatment and only mild to moderate dependence are also factors, as is a view of alcohol use as a bad habit rather than a disease. The fact that this is the case suggests that comorbidity is important to consider. As we know, comorbidity is the rule with adolescent substance abuse, raising questions about how effective an intervention MI might be with the typical adolescent seen in a psychiatric setting. Nonetheless, Battjes and colleagues (Battjes et al., 2004), using a manual-guided, group therapy format found MI to be effective in reducing marijuana use in a large sample of adolescent outpatients, although neither other substance abuse nor criminal behavior decreased in this group. Only modest effects were found in reducing smoking in adolescent psychiatric inpatients (Brown et al., 2003). On a more positive note, a small group (13) of inpatients, aged 18–35, with comorbid nonopioid drug abuse and psychosis reduced their drug use and maintained their gains over a 12 month period (Kavanagh et al., 2004).

Harm reduction aspects of MI

Harm reduction is one of the more interesting aspects of MI. The concept has to do with accepting a partial change in high risk behavior, with the idea that something is better than nothing. Harm reduction tends to be controversial as, for example, in the case of needle-exchange programs for addicts. Promoting condom use among adolescents is another example—critics are convinced these measures lead to more of the behavior that is undesirable in the first place. Advocates of harm reduction argue that the behavior is going to occur anyway, so we are better off making it safer. Harm reduction is used in MI as a way of encouraging patients who are involved in high-risk behavior and who might despair of being able to change the behavior completely, that they might realize more modest goals within their reach.

Typical harm reduction strategies with alcohol use include: (1) setting limits on alcohol consumption, and (2) increasing awareness of safe-driving levels and awareness of the effects of alcohol abuse (Bailey et al., 2004). Harm reduction may be a particularly salient approach for adolescents—much adolescent high-risk behavior is time limited and phase-specific anyway. The rationale is: If one can help the adolescent get through the teen years without serious harm he is likely to discontinue the behaviors as an adult. Obviously this is not the case for all adolescents who engage in high-risk behavior. Harm reduction has attracted much criticism from those who see it as encouraging the behavior it is designed to modify.

Parameters of MI

MI is usually administered in a single session. Duration of interviews averages about one and a half hours in research settings. Training of interviewers in reported studies has varied from 2 hours to 31 hours. Most studies use relatively untrained therapists. An on-line CME course is available (Etheridge, Sullivan, and Tanner, 2003; Institute of Medicine, 1990; Woodruff et al., 2001). A baseline evaluation can be done using the Readiness to Change Questionnaire (Rollnick, Heather, Gold, & Hall, 1992), a 12-item questionnaire based on Prochaska and DiClemente's stages of change model (1982).

MI seems to be effective as a stand-alone intervention—for some people. For others, whose impairment and duration of problem behavior is such that they need inpatient or residential treatment, detoxification, or other services besides counseling or therapy, MI has been considered a type of treatment induction. That is, it gets the interviewee thinking about what he needs to do and creates receptivity for further intervention.

MI can be considered a type of planned single-session psychotherapy, for whose efficacy there is considerable empirical support (Bloom, 1992; Slaff, 1995). Bloom identified the essential features of this approach as (1) the identification and focus on one issue; (2) an active stance on the part of the therapist (who should ask questions and listen but not lecture or exhort); (3) the imparting of relevant information; (4) assessing the patient's current level of self-awareness. He advised commenting on affect and making sure whatever interpretations were offered were acceptable to the patient. The goal, at the end of the session, is that the patient and therapist will have identified some aspect of the patient's cognitive or affective life that is below his or her awareness and is creating problems. A template is created for making changes. Single-session or other short term psychotherapy is facilitated by the presence of a crisis, which serves to increase motivation to change. Slaff gave several clinical examples in which patients did not return for a second session but made dramatic improvements. He also reviewed the literature on successful single-session interventions, which emphasized the importance of the readiness of the patient to make changes.

In Bloom's model, a follow-up is done by telephone to ascertain what changes have occurred as a result of the session. If the patient says she did not act on the recommendations, she is told that she can always do so later when she is ready.

One can see parallels with aspects of MI such as the focus on a single issue, the use of reflective listening, and the monitoring of readiness to change.

MI has been embraced as a technique that can be incorporated into primary health care settings. Given the fact that 20–30% of adults seen in these settings have problems with alcohol, it would indeed be a cost-effective primary or secondary prevention strategy if successful. A high proportion of adolescents seen in hospital emergency departments have drug- and-or alcohol-related medical problems, especially those seen after automobile accidents. This is another site where a brief intervention makes sense (Burke, O'Sullivan, and Vaughan, 2005; Gregor et al., 2003; Johnston, Rivara, Droesch, Dunn, & Copass, 2002; Kelly, Donovan, Chung, Cook, & Delbridge, 2004; Maio et al., 2000; Maio et al., 2005; Monti et al., 1999; Spirito et al., 2004). Another venue where it has been tried is college campuses, where binge drinking and alcohol-related problems are a major concern (Baer et al., 2001; Borsari and Carey, 2000; Collins, Carey, & Sliwinsky, 2002; Marlatt et al., 1998).

Interventions in such non-substance abuse treatment settings are termed opportunistic interventions. That is, a patient may come into the office (or clinic or emergency room) with an (ostensibly) unrelated presenting problem, but is discovered to have an alcohol use problem, and can be given a brief intervention for this. There is a counterpart for this with psychiatric practice, where comorbid alcohol and substance abuse are estimated to occur in upwards of 50% of patients seen in mental health settings (Grilo et al., 1995).

As with any intervention studied in research settings, transferability to real world settings is always a question. If, in fact, MI is most useful as an opportunistic intervention, research settings are not places where people are seen who just happen to have the targeted problem; rather they are selected for it. And, of course, the therapists are research staff and not real-world clinicians.

Conclusion

Adolescents who present to primary care settings, or who come to the attention of school personnel or emergency rooms, are seldom in the end-stage throes of addiction, making them ideal candidates for brief interventions. This is also true of those adolescents seen in outpatient psychotherapy whose substance abuse or other health-endangering behavior is not impairing them enough for them to need more intensive forms of treatment. Finally, for those adolescents seen in psychiatric settings who have problems that are not the primary reason for their mental health treatment, such as smoking or being overweight, MI offers the possibility for opportunistic interventions, which, if successful, could have a long term impact on health and quality of life.

MI is intriguing from a variety of standpoints. First, despite its apparent simplicity, it defies explanation. It gives the addict, who views himself as helpless in the face of his addiction, a new way of seeing himself as someone capable of change. Together with its companion, TMC, it stands in contrast to the many highly specific treatment modalities that have been developed in recent years. Yet, like CBT, IPT, and others, it has a good evidence base. It is a relatively "old" modality, hearkening back to the pioneering work of such early theorists as Carl Rogers. Information is presented to a patient by a nonjudgmental therapist who listens to the patient's point of view and conveys hope and optimism. It seems to revolve around the interpersonal relationship that is the core of the therapeutic process. And let's not forget the importance of empathy, long recognized as a crucial ingredient to all effective therapy. That sounds uncomplicated. Yet, it is also mysterious, perhaps it is because it speaks to the essence of human freedom, which is essentially unknowable, and human choice, which is essentially unpredictable. Isn't this always the case with good psychotherapy?

Appendix 10.A: Motivational Interviewing Techniques*

- Use open-ended questions.
  "Tell me about your drinking."
  "What concerns do you have about your drinking?"
  "How can I help you with your drinking?"
- Use reflective listening.
  "I hear you."
  "I'm accepting, not judging you."
  "Please say more."

- Use affirmative statements
"You are very courageous to be so revealing about this."
"You've accomplished a lot in a short time."
"I can understand why drinking feels good to you."
- Use summary statements.
"What you said is important. Let's talk about it ..."
- Elicit self-motivational statements—these statements fall into four categories.
  1. Problem recognition—"I never realized how much I am drinking." "Maybe I have been taking foolish risks."
  2. Expression of concern—"I am really worried about my grades and how alcohol may be affecting them."
  3. Intention to change—"I don't know how, but I want to try."
  4. Theme about Optimism—"I think I can do it. I am going to overcome this problem."

Additional points about motivational interviewing

1. The primary goal of MI is to resolve ambivalence and resistance and to move patients into a commitment to change their behavior.

Example

From: "I am not interested in reducing my alcohol use. I drink less than my friends." "I see no reason to change how much I drink. It is part of the college experience. I am not having problems so why should I cut down?"

To: "If I stop drinking I will feel better and maybe do better in school. However I am not sure what my friends will think. I am not sure how I can party and have fun if I don't drink so much."

To: "Maybe I do drink too much. I am willing to try to cut down. How much do you think it is safe for me to drink?"

2. Motivation to change is elicited from the student from within. It is not imposed from without. MI does not involve the use of external threats.

Provider statements not based on MI:

"If you don't stop drinking, you will be expelled."
"If you don't stop drinking, you will lose your job."
"If you don't stop drinking, you will never get into graduate school."
"If you don't stop drinking now, you will turn into an alcoholic."

3. In MI, the clinicians are not passive agents or mirrors. They direct and facilitate change with a number of methods. Clinicians utilize empathy,

summarization, reflective listening, and other techniques. MI is not 100% clinician-directed or 100% client-centered but, rather, someplace in between. It is meant to be interactive, with both sides giving and taking. In this way, it is similar to developing a relationship based on mutual respect, trust, and acceptance.

4. MI avoids arguments, coercion, and labels. While a therapist who is using MI techniques may not agree with a student, he/she respects the student's perspective. A counselor can disagree. For example:

Student: "Doc, I don't think I have a problem or need to cut down."
Provider: "John, I have to respectfully disagree. You had a serious accident after you were drinking. You are not doing well in your classes. Your girlfriend left you. I am not sure how serious things are, but I think you should consider how alcohol is contributing to these problems."

5. MI does not use negative comments.

*Adapted from the: National Institute on Alcohol Abuse and Alcoholism *College Drinking Prevention.* Accessed May 17, 2006, at http://www.collegedrinkingprevention.gov/NIAAACollegeMaterials/trainingmanual/module_4.aspx.

References

Aliotta, S. L., Vlasnik, J. J., & Delor, B. (2004), Enhancing adherence to long-term medical therapy: A new approach to assessing and treating patients. *Adv. Ther.*, 21:214–231.

Baer, J. S., Kivlahan, D. R., Blume, A. W., McKnight, P., & Marlatt, G. A. (2001), Brief intervention for heavy-drinking college students: 4-year follow-up and natural history. *Am. J. Public Health*, 91:1310–1316.

Bailey, K. A., Baker, A. L., Webster, R. A., & Lewin, T. J. (2004), Pilot randomized controlled trial of a brief alcohol intervention group for adolescents. *Drug Alcohol Rev.*, 23:157–166.

Battjes, R. J., Gordon, M. S., O'Grady, K. E., Kinlock, T. W., Katz, E. C., & Sears, E. A. (2004), Evaluation of a group-based substance abuse treatment program for adolescents. *J. Subst. Abuse Treat.*, 27:123–134.

Berg-Smith, S. M., Stevens, V. J., Brown, K. M., Van, H. L., Gernhofer, N., Peters, E., Greenberg, R., Snetselaar, L., Ahrens, L., & Smith, K. (1999), A brief motivational intervention to improve dietary adherence in adolescents: The Dietary Intervention Study in Children (DISC) Research Group. *Health Educ. Res.*, 14:399–410.

Bloom, B. L. (1992), *Planned Short-Term Psychotherapy.* Boston: Allyn & Bacon.

Boekeloo, B. O., Jerry, J., Lee-Ougo, W. I., Worrell, K. D., Hamburger, E. K., Russek-Cohen, E., & Snyder, M. H. (2004), Randomized trial of brief office-based interventions to reduce adolescent alcohol use. *Arch. Pediatr. Adolesc. Med.*, 158:635–642.

Borsari, B. & Carey, K. B. (2000), Effects of a brief motivational intervention with college student drinkers. *J. Consult Clin. Psychol.*, 68:728–733.

Breslin, C., Li, S., Sdao-Jarvie, K., Tupker, E., & Ittig-Deland, V. (2002), Brief treatment for young substance abusers: A pilot study in an addiction treatment setting. *Psychol. Addict. Behav.*, 16:10–16.

Brown, R. A., Ramsey, S. E., Strong, D. R., Myers, M. G., Kahler, C. W., Lejuez, C. W., Niaura, R., Pallonen, U. E., Kazura, A. N., Goldstein, M. G., & Abrams, D. B. (2003), Effects of motivational interviewing on smoking cessation in adolescents with psychiatric disorders. *Tob. Control* (12 Suppl 4) IV3–10.

Burke, P. J., O'Sullivan, J., & Vaughan, B. L. (2005), Adolescent substance use: Brief interventions by emergency care providers. *Pediatr. Emerg. Care*, 21:770–776.

Channon, S., Smith, V. J., & Gregory, J. W. (2003), A pilot study of motivational interviewing in adolescents with diabetes. *Arch. Dis. Child*, 88:680–683.

Collins, S. E., Carey, K. B., & Sliwinski, M. J. (2002), Mailed personalized normative feedback as a brief intervention for at-risk college drinkers. *J. Stud. Alcohol*, 63:559–567.

DiIorio, C., Resnicow, K., McDonnell, M., Soet, J., McCarty, F., & Yeager, K. (2003), Using motivational interviewing to promote adherence to antiretroviral medications: A pilot study. *J. Assoc. Nurses AIDS Care*, 14:52–62.

Edwards, G., Orford, J., Egert, S., Guthrie, S., Hawker, A., Hensman, C., Mitcheson, M., Oppenheimer, E., & Taylor, C. (1977), Alcoholism: A controlled trial of "treatment" and "advice." *J. Stud. Alcohol*, 38:1004–1031.

Etheridge, R. M., Sullivan, E., & Tanner, T. B. 2003. Brief interventions for alcohol use problems. Alcohol CME Curriculum. Available at http://www1.alcoholcme.com, accessed 5/17/06.

Gregor, M. A., Shope, J. T., Blow, F. C., Maio, R. F., Weber, J. E., & Nypaver, M. M. (2003), Feasibility of using an interactive laptop program in the emergency department to prevent alcohol misuse among adolescents. *Ann. Emerg. Med.*, 42:276–284.

Grilo, C. M., Becker, D. F., Walker, M. L., Levy, K. N., Edell, W. S., & McGlashan, T. H. (1995), Psychiatric comorbidity in adolescent inpatients with substance use disorders. *J. Amer. Acad. Child Adolesc. Psychiat.*, 34:1085–1091.

Hungerford, D. W., Williams, J. M., Furbee, P. M., Manley, W. G., III, Helmkamp, J. C., Horn, K., & Pollock, D. A. (2003), Feasibility of screening and intervention for alcohol problems among young adults in the ED. *Am. J. Emerg. Med.*, 21:14–22.

Institute of Medicine (1990), *Broadening the Base of Treatment for Alcohol Problems.* Washington, DC: National Academy Press.

Johnston, B. D., Rivara, F. P., Droesch, R. M., Dunn, C., & Copass, M. K. (2002), Behavior change counseling in the emergency department to reduce injury risk: A randomized, controlled trial. *Pediatrics*, 110:267–274.

Kavanagh, D. J., Young, R., White, A., Saunders, J. B., Wallis, J., Shockley, N., Jenner, L., & Clair, A. (2004), A brief motivational intervention for substance misuse in recent-onset psychosis. *Drug Alcohol Rev.*, 23:151–155.

Kelly, T. M., Donovan, J. E., Chung, T., Cook, R. L., & Delbridge, T. R. (2004), Alcohol use disorders among emergency department-treated older adolescents: A new brief screen (RUFT-Cut) using the AUDIT, CAGE, CRAFFT, and RAPS-QF. *Alcohol Clin. Exp. Res.*, 28:746–753.

Kirk, S., Scott, B. J., & Daniels, S. R. (2005), Pediatric obesity epidemic: Treatment options. *J. Am. Diet. Assoc.*, 105:S44-S51.

Larimer, M. E., Turner, A. P., Anderson, B. K., Fader, J. S., Kilmer, J. R., Palmer, R. S., & Cronce, J. M. (2001), Evaluating a brief alcohol intervention with fraternities. *J. Stud. Alcohol*, 62:370–380.

Levy, S., Vaughan, B. L., & Knight, J. R. (2002), Office-based intervention for adolescent substance abuse. *Pediatr. Clin. North Am.*, 49:329–343.

Maio, R. F., Shope, J. T., Blow, F. C., Copeland, L. A., Gregor, M. A., Brockmann, L. M., Weber, J. E., & Metrou, M. E. (2000), Adolescent injury in the emergency department: Opportunity for alcohol interventions? *Ann. Emerg. Med.*, 35:252–257.

Maio, R. F., Shope, J. T., Blow, F. C., Gregor, M. A., Zakrajsek, J. S., Weber, J. E., & Nypaver, M. M. (2005), A randomized controlled trial of an emergency department-based interactive computer program to prevent alcohol misuse among injured adolescents. *Ann. Emerg. Med.*, 45:420–429.

Marlatt, G. A., Baer, J. S., Kivlahan, D. R., Dimeff, L. A., Larimer, M. E., Quigley, L. A., Somers, J. M., & Williams, E. (1998), Screening and brief intervention for high-risk college student drinkers: Results from a 2-year follow-up assessment. *J. Consult Clin. Psychol.*, 66:604–615.

Miller, W. R. (1996), Motivational interviewing: Research, practice, and puzzles. *Addict. Behav.*, 21:835–842.

Monti, P. M., Colby, S. M., Barnett, N. P., Spirito, A., Rohsenow, D. J., Myers, M., Woolard, R., & Lewander, W. (1999), Brief intervention for harm reduction with alcohol-positive older adolescents in a hospital emergency department. *J. Consult Clin. Psychol.*, 67:989–994.

Prochaska, J. O. & DiClemente, C. C. (1982), Transtheoretical therapy: Toward a more integrative model of change. *Psychotherapy: Theory, Research and Practice*, 19:276–287.

Rollnick, S., Heather, N., Gold, R., & Hall, W. (1992), Development of a short "readiness to change" questionnaire for use in brief, opportunistic interventions among excessive drinkers. *Br. J. Addict.*, 87:743–754.

Rosner, R. (2005), The scourge of addiction: What the adolescent psychiatrist needs to know. *Adolescent Psychiatry*, 29:19–31.

Skaret, E., Weinstein, P., Kvale, G., & Raadal, M. (2003), An intervention program to reduce dental avoidance behaviour among adolescents: A pilot study. *Eur. J. Paediatr. Dent.*, 4:191–196.

Slaff, B. (1995), Thoughts on short-term and single-session therapy. *Adolescent Psychiatry*, 20:299–306.

Spirito, A., Monti, P. M., Barnett, N. P., Colby, S. M., Sindelar, H., Rohsenow, D. J., Lewander, W., & Myers, M. (2004), A randomized clinical trial of a brief motivational intervention for alcohol-positive adolescents treated in an emergency department. *J. Pediatr.*, 145:396–402.

Spoth, R. L., Redmond, C., & Shin, C. (2001), Randomized trial of brief family interventions for general populations: Adolescent substance use outcomes 4 years following baseline. *J. Consult Clin. Psychol.*, 69:627–642.

Stewart, S. H., Conrod, P. J., Marlatt, G. A., Comeau, M. N., Thush, C., & Krank, M. (2005), New developments in prevention and early intervention for alcohol abuse in youths. *Alcohol Clin. Exp. Res.*, 29:278–286.

Tait, R. J. & Hulse, G. K. (2003), A systematic review of the effectiveness of brief interventions with substance using adolescents by type of drug. *Drug Alcohol Rev.*, 22:337–346.

Tait, R. J. & Hulse, G. K. (2005), Adolescent substance use and hospital presentations: A record linkage assessment of 12-month outcomes. *Drug Alcohol Depend.*, 79:365–371.

Tevyaw, T. O. & Monti, P. M. (2004), Motivational enhancement and other brief interventions for adolescent substance abuse: Foundations, applications and evaluations. *Addiction*, 99 (Suppl 2):63–75.

Woodruff, S. I., Edwards, C. C., Conway, T. L., & Elliott, S. P. (2001), Pilot test of an Internet virtual world chat room for rural teen smokers. *J. Adolesc. Health*, 29:239–243.

11 Adolescent choice in disputed custody
The role of the forensic psychiatric consultant

Harvey Feinberg, M.D.

Abstract

This chapter reviews the history of legal decision-making in child custody, showing how the role of an expert in forensic psychiatry has come to play an increasingly important role. Although adolescents' preferences with respect to custody and visitation are generally given considerable weight, they are only one of many factors that guide the courts in making decisions. A psychiatrist with expertise in evaluating adolescents and providing consultation to judges can play an important role in helping the courts make decisions that are in the best interests of the adolescent. Numerous case examples are presented to illustrate the work of the psychiatrist who acts as a forensic consultant.

Introduction

Divorcing spouses today contest few issues more bitterly than child custody. This was not always the case. When a married couple petitioned the courts of ancient Rome for a divorce, any disputes over which parent would retain primary physical custody of the children were easily settled. They were easily settled because there were no disputes. In the eyes of Caesar's jurists, children were property owned solely by their fathers. The legal rights of mothers were limited since the courts also considered them to be the property of their husbands.

The practice of automatically granting fathers primary physical custody in all but the rarest cases spread around the world and continued well into the 19th century. Under English common law in the 1800s, this practice became virtually self-perpetuating. Though judges could find for the mother in custody disputes, this rarely happened, due to property laws which decreed that once a man lost title to his assets—in this case his children—his financial responsibility for them also ended. Since few women of that time possessed the resources to support a family on their own, the courts remained averse to awarding custody to the mother even if the children stated a strong preference for living with her.

The tender years doctrine

A gradual shift in custody decisions occurred as the courts entered the 20th century. Historical trends such as the Industrial Revolution forced a division of family responsibilities, thrusting fathers away from the family home and into roles as wage earners, while mothers stayed behind as caretakers to the children. This division of roles, as well as an increasing interest in children's welfare, led to a shift from paternal preference to maternal preference in custody decisions. The tender years doctrine suggested that children under the age of 10 could not attain normal emotional development without the continual influence of a maternal presence. By the 1920s, tender years became the standard in 48 states. Over time, it became the father who seldom retained custody of the children, even if the children were adolescents and presumably beyond the consideration of any tender years' standard.

A judicial shift

Feminism and the gender politics that marked the late 1960s and early 1970s inspired a further shift in custody decisions. As women attained greater equality in the workplace, with a subsequent increase in duties, traditional parenting roles expanded and diversified. Many fathers assumed greater responsibility for the daily upbringing of the children. In some households, mothers became the primary breadwinners while fathers stayed home caring for the family. The term "househusband" entered the lexicon.

As men demonstrated parenting skills comparable to women, judges became less reluctant to award custodial rights to fathers. Fathers began to seek primary custody more often, at times even claiming sex discrimination in custody proceedings. Gradually, court rulings and statutory guidelines awarded more rights to fathers. In a landmark decision in 1981 in the case of *Devine vs. Devine*, the Alabama court asserted that the tender years doctrine represented a form of gender bias against men and violated the Fourteenth Amendment by denying fathers "the equal protection of the law."

By the 1970s, most states had substituted the tender years doctrine with the "best interests of the child" standard. This standard compelled jurists to award custody based on what is best for the child considering the particular circumstances, rather than simply the gender of the parent. The acceptance of the best interests standard led the way to the development of joint custody in divorce proceedings. Parents argued that it was in the best interest of the children to have access to and rearing from both parents. Child welfare experts began to uncover evidence that access to both parents is critical to a child's self-esteem and coping (Lewis, 1978; Derdeyn and Scott, 1984; American Psychological Association, 1994; Ackerman and Ackerman, 1997; Herman, 1997). In 1979, California became the first state to enact a joint custody statute. At this time, nearly all states have adopted joint custody statutes or recognize the concept of joint custody in case law.

Unlike the tender years standard, in which judges need only apply a rule, the best interests standard is more difficult for judges because the decision is less obvious. They must sift through a great deal of information and are often torn between two seemingly capable parents. Therefore, since the introduction of the best interests standard and the ensuing popularity of joint custody arrangements, forensic psychiatrists have played an increasingly prominent role in helping the court to determine the best custody arrangement. In a 1992 study of 282 disputed custody cases, Kunin, Ebbesen, and Konecni (1992) found that only two factors directly impacted the judges' decisions: child preference and the recommendations of the forensic consultant.

Adolescent choice in disputed custody

Although adolescents' preferences regarding which parent with whom they live are likely to be given greater weight by courts than are the wishes of young children, they do not have complete freedom to decide (Speth, 1995). Even in states in which the law specifically allows adolescents to choose the parent with whom they wish to live, a forensic psychiatrist can fulfill a critical role in helping the court to render a decision. For example, Ohio law empowers the judge to award custody to the parent chosen by the adolescent "unless the court finds...that it would not be in the best interest of the child to have the choice" (Ohio Revised Code, Annotated, Section 3109.4).

Many other jurisdictions have similar guidelines that require the judge to ascertain whether the adolescent is competent enough to express a reasoned preference. Additionally, it is critical to examine the adolescent's underlying motivations for choosing a particular caretaker. An adolescent may be motivated by such simple factors as the leniency of one parent compared to the other or by more complex factors such as alienation or loyalty conflict. It is the forensic consultant who can provide, through interviews and data gathering, a "valid and reliable assessment of the child's preference, the reasoning for the preference, and the quality of the relationship with her respective parents" (Levy, 1986).

The role of the forensic psychiatrist

As Kunin, Ebbesen, and Konecni have indicated (1992), the information gathered in a forensic psychiatrist's interviews may heavily influence a judge's decision. If the expert has been appointed by the court—rather than hired by one of the opposing sides in the custody dispute—judges will frequently follow the consultant's conclusion (Haller, 1981; Clark, 1995).

However, some judges I have spoken with do not want psychiatrists to make recommendations regarding which parent should retain custody. Rather, they are looking for "a factual flow of information" that cannot be directly obtained by the court—information that can be gathered through such means as home visits, obtaining access to school records, and observing parent/adolescent interactions.

As one prominent New York jurist said, "I want a forensic [consultant] to do what I can't do, which is, get off that bench, visit them...provide me with as much information as possible." Another judge I spoke with took that thought a bit further: "I think the forensic's got to be a bit of a sleuth...because the forensic has got to find the information and make it click...sift through and present it and make an assessment as to where the veracity is, at least in the forensic's mind, that would assist the judge."

Determining which parent will better serve the adolescent's best interests presents a challenge quite apart from making the same determination for a preadolescent child. The forensic educator must first consider the tasks adolescents confront, including:

- Coping effectively with aggressive and sexual drives
- Developing a stable ego and sexual identity
- Establishing a stable moral code
- Developing ego autonomy
- Appropriate separation and individuation
- Vocational choice
- Sexual object choice

These tasks create formidable stresses for the developing adolescent that preadolescent children do not encounter. The parent who retains primary physical custody must therefore possess the skills to properly respond to these stresses and facilitate the adolescent's mastering of these tasks. Custodial parents will be called upon to manage fluctuating emotions and attendant acts of aggressiveness and rebellion (Wallerstein and Kelly, 1996; Wallerstein, Lewis, and Blakeslee, 2000). They must also be prepared to cope with that inevitable day when the adolescent starts to flex his or her independence and to break away from the parental bonds until the parent is no longer the primary object of affection.

During that period, the adolescent will waver in his or her affection, vacillating between clinging to the primary object of affection and fighting to free himself/herself from that object (Schwartzberg, 1980; 1981). The custodial parent must have the emotional stability to tolerate such conflicts while supporting the adolescent's quest for independence. It is during the interview process that the psychiatrist must uncover the adolescent's emotional requirements and match them against each parent's ability to meet them.

Making the correct determination is a crucial step towards protecting the adolescent's best interest. In their detailed study of 21 adolescents from divorced families, Wallerstein and Kelly (1974) found that divorce "poses a very specific hazard to the normal adolescent process of emancipation from primary love objects." Essentially, the divorce can either interrupt an adolescent's entry into adulthood or accelerate it. Three major psychopathological formations may develop as a consequence: prolonged interference with advancement into adulthood, temporary interference with this advancement, or pseudoadvancement.

Collecting the data

In a typical custody case, the psychiatrist will conduct three to four interviews with the adolescent. Ideally, the evaluator should meet with the adolescent on his or her own two or three times, with one of the interviews conducted in the adolescent's home. I interview the adolescent once with the mother and once with the father so I can observe how he or she interacts with each parent. I also meet with each parent separately without the adolescent present to obtain each parent's history as well as the developmental history of the adolescent.

The forensic psychiatrist should conduct a school visit to interview the adolescent's guidance counselor and primary teachers as well as the principal, where available. I ask them to share their evaluations of the adolescent's social skills, developmental level, cognitive reasoning, and emotional intelligence. They might also lend some insight into the adolescent's relationship with both parents.

The consultant can chart fluctuations in an adolescent's emotions by examining school records for declines in academic performance or behavior. School records can also corroborate or refute other data. For example, a father reported that his 16-year old son often seemed inhibited, troubled, and withdrawn when they were together. In contrast, a recent school report had indicated that the boy was outgoing with his peers and possessed highly developed social skills. He served as captain on the school's debating team, a position ill suited for a withdrawn individual. The contrast in his behavior in two different settings suggested that the boy's behavior with his father may have represented a reaction to their relationship. Further interviews with the father and son provided an opportunity to further develop such data.

If the adolescent or either parent is undergoing therapy, I request permission to interview the therapist. However, the information obtained from the therapist may be rather limited since mental health professionals, bound as they are by confidentiality constraints, are usually guarded when speaking about their clients and most will refrain from revealing a diagnosis.

I also interview any members of the extended family who live with the adolescent, as well as others who are involved with her life, such as nannies and tutors. It is important to bear in mind that these people will naturally have biases towards the spouse they are related to or employed by. For instance, a paternal grandfather will rarely criticize the manner in which his son raises his own family, especially considering such criticism will be recorded. Grandparents have a vested interest in ensuring that their own child retains custody of the grandchildren. Nannies and tutors are paid employees who, for the most part, feel compelled to remain loyal to whichever spouse pays them.

First contact

The challenge in a custody evaluation is to build, in only a few sessions, some semblance of the kind of relationship which often requires months for a psychiatrist and patient to form in therapy. The purpose of the interviews is to collect information, unlike the situation in therapy where the therapist's primary role is to help the patient. The challenge for a forensic psychiatrist is to quickly create the bond of empathy and trust that inspires open, honest communication, without holding out the prospect of alleviating suffering, as would be the case in therapy.

The psychiatrist should open the interview by describing his or her role in the custody process to the adolescent, even though the parents have probably already explained this. I begin by identifying myself as a court-appointed professional who has been charged with gathering information that will help the judge determine which parent will retain custody. It is important that adolescents understand that I may report anything they disclose during our sessions and that these observations may determine their living conditions for some time to come.

My preference is to conduct the first interview with the adolescent in my office, and the second interview in his or her home. The home environment usually offers many clues pertaining to the adolescent's personality. This is especially true of the teenager's room, which is where I prefer to do the interview. The moment I walk into an adolescent's room, my eyes search for those clues. I want to know what books the adolescent reads, what activities and hobbies he or she engages in. I am looking for information that will suggest a line of questioning as the interview develops. That information will also allow me to introduce subjects with which the adolescent is familiar—such as a favorite sport or hobby—thus facilitating dialogue by putting the adolescent at ease.

The observations a forensic psychiatrist initially makes during a home visit can also provide the means for quickly drawing out the adolescent. The following case examples illustrate this. (The names and identifying information of all the adolescents have been changed.)

Case example #1

Emily* was a fourteen-year-old whose bedroom bookshelf contained books on the Rosenberg trial. I learned that the case fascinated her. She had extensively studied it in her high school history class and had written several reports on the verdict. During a discussion of the trial, she disclosed her thoughts on right and wrong, innocence and guilt, and justice and fairness. She even expressed opinions on how the American judicial system worked. As she spoke, I observed her cognitive reasoning, emotional feelings, and level of maturity, which was far advanced

---

* Denotes a name change.

for her age. That information gave me some idea of the skills a custodial parent would need to help further her cognitive and emotional maturity.

Case example #2

When I met with Michael, a twelve-year-old, in the living room of his mother's apartment, one of the first things I noticed was an ornate chess set opened on a coffee table. I also noticed several books about chess sitting on the desk in his bedroom. At the start of the interview, Michael acted withdrawn. I asked him the questions I put to all adolescents during this process, inviting him to share his feelings about his peers and teachers, his neighborhood and school. I asked him the names of his friends and what they did when they spent time together.

Michael restricted himself to short answers that revealed very little about his personality or feelings. But when I referred to the chess set and asked if he played, Michael replied with heightened enthusiasm. He carried in the set and proudly showed me each of the intricately cut pieces. We talked about the game at some length. During that discussion Michael demonstrated a sophistication and intelligence beyond that of a typical twelve-year-old. I returned to the questions about his academic and social life and this time he spoke much more candidly about his feelings.

To gain insight into his relationship with his parents, I asked whether he played chess with them and he replied, "My dad gave me the set. He plays with me whenever I see him." Michael went on to demonstrate some of the chess strategies his father had taught him. As he described the games he had played against his father, Michael's manner was bubbly and engaged. His memories of those matches were obviously pleasurable. When I asked Michael if his mother ever played chess with him, his demeanor changed. His voice lowered into a monotone. "She doesn't play chess," he said. I asked in which activities he and his mother participated when they spent time together. "She goes out a lot with her boyfriend," he replied. "I like him but he takes up too much of her time."

I invited Michael to provide an example and he told me of an incident that had occurred three months earlier. He had entered a local hospital for a minor operation. His mother had accompanied him to the hospital and took him home after the procedure. Then she went out for the evening, leaving Michael in the care of his maternal grandmother. Sometime during the night Michael experienced pain and discomfort, common reactions to the operation he had undergone, but still alarming for a twelve-year-old boy. He placed numerous phone calls trying to locate his mother without success. Michael finally called his father who immediately came over and spent the night with his son.

By the time Michael finished relating this story, he was no longer speaking in a monotone. His voice sounded distant and pained. His eyes were tearing. He agreed to repeat what he had told me when we met for the joint interview with his mother. She admitted that she had kept a dinner engagement that evening but expressed surprise that her absence had disturbed her son. She explained that the doctors had assured her that the procedure posed no danger to Michael, and the grandmother was left to stay with him, so she assumed her presence after the operation was, to use her words, "not necessary."

She could not, however, explain why she had neglected to leave a phone number where she could be reached if any complications arose. She could not explain why she had not told her son in advance that she would be gone for the evening. Her behavior in this matter led me to ask other questions that revealed a mother who, at the time, was self-absorbed and lacking in empathy. However, she did become much more involved in his life as the divorce proceedings continued. This is not uncommon. Custody disputes often activate the dormant interests of parents who have been previously distant.

In my interview with the father, he impressed me as being engaged with many aspects of Michael's life and interested in his welfare. Subsequent interviews with Michael's teachers corroborated this evaluation.

In this particular case, my final report included a recommendation that the father, on the basis of his reliability, consistency, and parenting skills, should retain custody of Michael with liberal visitation for the mother. The judge concurred with this finding, one that would have been difficult to reach had I been unable to begin a meaningful dialogue with Michael. By noticing the objects in the adolescent's home and using them to facilitate conversation, I was able to establish rapport with Michael, and he felt more comfortable opening up to me, a tactic that I often use and that I certainly recommend.

When the adolescent articulates a preference

Over the course of the second interview, Michael had expressed so much animosity towards his mother that it was obvious, without asking him, which parent he would prefer to live with. His strong preference for his father did influence my final report. It is, however, not a question I often ask outright. A judge might appropriately pose that question to an adolescent during an in camera interview in his chambers, but I think it best for the psychiatrist performing an evaluation to refrain from asking the adolescent to articulate a choice. In many cases, the adolescent's reply will be too ambiguous to be of much help. There also is the risk that the question may arouse feelings of hostility, helplessness, and loyalty conflict, causing the adolescent to emotionally withdraw and become less forthcoming with the interviewer. The question might even trigger an antagonism that can linger into subsequent interviews and undermine the evaluation process.

Even when an adolescent voluntarily states a preference, the forensic consultant must still ascertain the underlying motivations for the choice and whether that choice truly represents the adolescent's best interests, as illustrated in the following vignette.

Case example #3

During my second interview with him, Daniel*, a fifteen-year-old, volunteered insistently that he wished to stay with his mother, but declined to state any reasons for his preference.

As we spoke about his relationship with his mother, a picture formed of a woman who was transforming her son into a replacement for an absent husband. She frequently asked Daniel for approval of her physical appearance and dress. She would confide in him about matters that would be more appropriately discussed with an adult peer, such as dating and her own feelings about the divorce.

His mother told me that Daniel frequently issued orders to her—behavior she referred to as "cute" and "normal for a growing boy." An examination of his school records revealed that Daniel had recently expressed belligerence towards his teachers and schoolmates. He had instigated two fist fights and was currently serving an extended probation. This behavior ordinarily would have meant expulsion, but as Daniel had received exemplary grades in behavior throughout his school career, both the schoolmaster and guidance counselor considered his recent behavior a reaction to the divorce proceedings and an aberration.

During our last interview, I asked Daniel how he felt about being the "man of the house." He hesitated before answering, but finally admitted that he felt uncomfortable with the role his mother had imposed on him. Yet he had never voiced any objections to her. He had come to believe that his mother needed his protection, as inadequate as it might be.

I asked what would happen if he no longer lived with her full time. He couldn't articulate a specific outcome. However he seemed certain that she would have difficulty functioning without his continual presence in the home. "My father has a girlfriend," Daniel explained, "My mother has no one but me to take care of her."

It is not uncommon for some adolescents to assume a role of caretaker for a dysfunctional parent, particularly in a mother-son relationship. The danger in the example with Daniel is that the mother's behavior had forced him to assume a level of adulthood for which he was unprepared. Tooley (1976) describes how this blurring of generational boundaries causes feelings of anxiety and guilt for the adolescent. To defend against these feelings, the adolescent often resorts to acting-out and aggressive behavior, as in Daniel's case. In some cases, this blurring of boundaries leads to role reversal, which, if prolonged, can lead to a pseudo-adult stance that denies age appropriate dependency needs and can interfere with development.

I was very concerned about the effects that the caretaker role Daniel had accepted in his relationship with his mother would impose on him, both in the short term and the long term. Daniel's father had impressed me as someone who could discipline his son without obstructing the boy's search for independence. Despite Daniel's preference, I recommended that the court award custody to the father with liberal visitation for the mother. I have subsequently learned that Daniel has thrived under

---

* Denotes a name change.

this arrangement and that his mother, who entered therapy shortly after the divorce decree was granted, is also moving towards her own independence.

Alienation

When an adolescent voluntarily articulates a strong preference, the forensic psychiatrist should consider whether he or she may have been subject to alienation (Gardner, 1988; Johnston, 2003). This is a controversial issue. Many judges refrain from basing their decisions on alienation because the charge is very difficult to prove and becomes a hotly contested issue in court.

Some of the clues are subtle, but others are extremely obvious. Alienation can be so achieved that the adolescent will not admit or, in some cases, even be consciously aware that one parent has manipulated his or her attitude towards the other parent. Since judges encounter difficulty interpreting the signs of alienation, they turn to the forensic for guidance. As one jurist revealed, "How can I ascertain whether an adolescent has been, in effect, brainwashed? I don't have the skills to make that determination, certainly not on the basis of a single interview in my chambers. The adolescent says he loves his mother and hates his father. How can you prove otherwise when the father charges alienation? That's the kind of case where we look to the forensic to provide insight into the past and current family dynamic."

In one custody case, I investigated an alienation charge brought by the father. The two children, a twelve-year-old boy and fourteen-year-old girl, had refused to spend any time with him. Whenever he arrived to pick them up for a visit, the adolescents claimed that they were too ill or simply refused to go. On the rare occasions when the children did visit his home, they spent an inordinate amount of time on the phone with their mother.

During our initial interview, both children acted sullen and rude. Neither child would say anything positive about the father. When asked why they refused to spend time with him, they replied that the father's visitations were disruptive, that he always picked days when they had more attractive activities to pursue in school or with friends. I explained to them that their father had no choice; he was following the schedule the judge had recommended. The daughter replied, "He just doesn't care how he upsets our lives."

The adolescents claimed that they didn't like the activities their father chose when they did go out together. "Movie, museums and restaurants," his son complained, "he never takes us anywhere fun." I asked the boy where he would like his father to take them. "I don't want to go anywhere with him ever," he replied.

I asked the children to specify what they disliked about their father. They said he didn't feed them properly and that he was quick to anger. They accused him of failing to financially support the family. "When our TV was broken," the girl said, "it took Dad weeks to pay the repair bill." She went on to complain that the father was going to sell property that had been in the family for years. I asked why she would hang up the phone on her father whenever he called. She replied, "I want to show him what it's like when he hangs up on mommy."

The boy described his father as uncommunicative, physically abusive, and subject to abrupt mood swings. "I never know when he's going to fly off the handle," he said. He expressed hostility towards his father's girlfriend and ridiculed her for being overweight. At one point, he called the father a liar. On the other hand, both children had nothing but praise for their mother.

All of these complaints could have been true. However, after interviewing both parents, the children's therapist, and the representative of the school, as well as reviewing the school records, I concluded that the mother may well have alienated the children. I based my conclusion on the following indicators:

- The children had parroted the same complaints against the father that the mother had articulated during my interview with her. All three of them had used many of the same phrases—including "fly off the handle"—to describe the father's behavior.
- The mother insisted that the father pick up the children in the lobby of their apartment building rather than in their apartment. The children had interpreted this to mean that the father was a man to be feared and ostracized.
- There were no records to support the mother and children's claim that the father was physically abusive. The children's therapist said that neither the boy nor the girl had ever complained about abuse. The mother had never petitioned the family court for an order of protection or reported any abuse to the Administration of Children's Services.
- The complaints, such as the sale of the property and the tardy payment of the repair bill, reflected the mother's concerns more than the children's. The property was an undeveloped tract that the children had never visited. It seemed unlikely that they could have developed an emotional attachment to land they had never seen. The mother, however, had vehemently opposed its sale.
- The mother would often have one of the children call the father to ask whether he had paid the most recent bills, an act that reinforced that notion that the father was not adequately providing for the family.
- There was evidence that the children had both expressed affection for their father at the start of the divorce proceedings. Their therapist's notes indicated that she had observed them enjoying their time with him. The notes also confirmed that the children first presented a great deal of anger towards the father while they were in their mother's care, well after the divorce proceedings had commenced.
- The father had shown me over a dozen photographs depicting him and the children on vacation shortly before the divorce came to trial. In the photos, they appeared outwardly affectionate and pleased to be in his presence.

- Testimony from disinterested third parties indicated the mother had repeatedly denigrated the father in front of the children. In my own interviews with her, the mother never uttered a single positive word about him.

In the end, the children decided this issue. Before my evaluation was completed, they both suffered a severe depression requiring hospitalization on a psychiatric unit. The children continued to avoid seeing their father except on an extremely limited basis. The court had no alternative but to accept the children's wishes to remain with their mother.

The judge did grant liberal visitation to the father in the hopes that he could repair the breach with his children. I learned in later years that reconciliation never took place. The children steadfastly refused to see their father except on rare occasions. He remarried and they gradually drifted further apart until there was no contact between them.

The other side of alienation

After a spouse charges alienation, the task for the forensic is to determine whether the adolescent's hostility is the product of alienation, a reaction to poor parenting, or a combination of both. An example is a case a judge assigned to me in which the father claimed the mother had marginalized his relationship with their fourteen-year-old daughter Alicia.*

As part of the complaint, the father's attorney wrote that Alicia had been "... programmed to an extent that we interpret as a form of child abuse." He went further to say that the mother had not cooperated in encouraging the daughter to have a positive relationship with her father and that the mother had made her daughter so emotionally dependent on her that the daughter became convinced that only the mother could provide her with emotional sustenance.

Alicia opened our initial interview by declaring, "If I have to stay with my father, my life will be over." I asked her why she felt that way. She replied, "My father never lets my friends come to the house," she said, "He pulls me around by the wrist so hard it hurts. If I say anything nice about mom, he gets angry. He uses curse words when he talks about her and he won't let me call her when I'm with him. He calls me an idiot whenever I make a mistake. He screams over the littlest things. He never asks me how I'm doing in school or if I need anything. He forgets to make lunch for me. He just doesn't care. I think the only reason he wants me is to make mom mad." Alicia insisted that she could not stand to be in his presence, not even for short visitations. She had nothing positive to say about him.

Alicia's response sounded spontaneous; it revealed none of the "laundry list" qualities common to coached testimony. Parroting was also notably absent. Her complaints against her father reflected his emotional neglect or insensitivity towards her needs. A visit to Alicia's school partially corroborated her claim that

---

* Denotes a name change.

her father took scant interest in her studies. The principal and her teachers could recall having met him only once or twice in three years. All of them were familiar with Alicia's mother.

When I interviewed the father, he insisted that he had always taken an interest in Alicia's schoolwork. But he could only name one of her teachers and could not identify her best and worst subjects. He denied pulling Alicia's wrist or using profanity in her presence. He claimed he yelled at her only "when she gets out of line." He said he had no difficulty with anger management. However, when I related what his daughter had said about him, he underwent a transformation. He clenched his teeth and his face became slightly colored. When he finally spoke, his words were measured but his tone was almost surly. He resembled a volcano resisting eruption, though he quickly composed himself.

The father said he did not allow Alicia's friends to visit his home because they were "part of a bad crowd" and he was trying to discourage her from seeing them for "her own well-being." Yet, during a school visit a guidance counselor had told me that Alicia's closest friends were among the school's top students and that her own record of behavior was excellent.

The father dismissed Alicia's claim that he often forgot to feed her by saying, "I eat on a crazy schedule and she's not used to it." He said he did not allow Alicia to call her mother because that would "take away from my time with her." I asked him to discuss his feelings about his wife. He replied, "I'd rather not."

When I spoke with the mother, she offered a balanced perspective of her husband's virtues as well as his shortcomings. She made no attempt to demonize him. Her portrayal of him was consistent with what Alicia had said when she had described her mother's feelings about her father.

I will often ask adolescents to project their future into the next two, five, and ten years in order to measure their developmental level and discover their interests. Those interests can then be matched against each parent's ability to nurture and develop them.

When I asked Alicia to project her future, she expressed a desire to become an attorney. Her mother had already compiled a list of law schools for Alicia to consider. She had given her daughter digital videorecordings of four courtroom dramas as Christmas presents and she had accompanied Alicia to several trials at the local courthouse. The father's gifts and visitation activities failed to demonstrate a similar insight into his daughter's interests.

After reviewing all the evidence, I concluded in my report that the mother had not alienated Alicia against her father, but that her antagonism toward him was due to the fact that he lacked the parental skills needed to develop a relationship with his daughter. Essentially, I concluded that Alicia's feeling were entirely her own, a reaction to poor parenting rather than alienation. The court rejected the father's claim of alienation and awarded custody to the mother.

Tending developmental needs

Adolescents must shed their childhood dependency on their parents if they are to establish an identity and attain full emotional maturity. Determining which parent can best facilitate this progress towards autonomy is one of the forensic consultant's primary tasks. This is true even if the adolescent presents signs of resisting independence, as the following case vignette illustrates.

Case example #4

Scott*, a thirteen-year-old, expressed affection for both of his parents in our first interview. He admitted to feelings of conflict over which parent should retain primary physical custody, while stating a preference for living with his mother. All of the evidence indicated that his mother and father were devoted to him. Despite both parents' obvious interest in Scott's welfare, their divorce had become very acrimonious, particularly on the mother's part. She wanted to retain custody of her son and had requested limited visitations for the father.

I interviewed Scott once with each parent. He appeared to be equally comfortable with each of them, though I saw more evidence of mutual empathy when he was with his mother. They listened to one another and would frequently laugh together. During my second interview with Scott, I asked him what he would like to change about his parents. He once again expressed loyalty to both of them but complained that his mother made him wear a helmet whenever he rode his bicycle. "It makes me look so dumb," Scott said, "and I know everybody's laughing at me when I have it on." I suggested that his mother insisted on the helmet to protect him against injury. "I know that," he replied, "but none of my friends have to wear helmets. She protects me too much."

He revealed that his mother accompanied him to school every morning, even though he was thirteen and they lived only six blocks from the building. She discouraged him from participating in sports by claiming they were too dangerous. She expressed apprehension when Scott visited his father on alternate weekends because her husband allowed him to sleep unaccompanied in a backyard tent on warm nights. She feared for the boy's safety even though the home was in a well-to-do, densely populated suburb with little crime. There certainly was hostility in Scott towards his mother over these impositions, but he was wary of expressing this to her.

I interviewed the mother alone and discovered that she was a cautious woman who took pains to avoid risks. I asked why she had insisted that a nanny accompany Scott and his father when they traveled on vacation. "I just don't think," she explained to me, "that his father will watch out for him as well as the nanny." The court totally disagreed and rejected her request.

---

* Denotes a name change.

This mother demonstrated no awareness that her over-protectiveness could damage Scott's self-esteem at a time when he should be moving towards independence. Her behavior was only prolonging Scott's latency period. When I asked him to project his future, his answers indicated a reluctance to accept positions of responsibility. Unlike other typical boys his age, he showed little interest in forming attachments that would threaten his relationship with his mother. He could not imagine growing up to live in a different town than she.

Despite her over-protective nature, the mother had demonstrated other sound parenting and communication skills. For example, Scott's teachers had praised her attentiveness to his academic career. The school's guidance counselor had noted that the father took a more permissive attitude towards his son's upbringing. Although he had enjoyed a warm relationship with Scott, the father had difficulty enforcing even the lightest discipline.

This was one of those cases in which the judge did not want a recommendation—just the facts. I wrote a report that summarized the collected data without a recommendation. However, I also emphasized the inherent dangers of impeding an adolescent's emotional growth. The judge granted primary physical custody to the mother but allowed alternate Friday to Monday morning visitations to the father, including regular weekly overnights and vacations without supervision and the sphere of extracurricular activities. His decision struck a balance that reconciled Scott's need for definable boundaries while safeguarding the adolescent's advancement towards autonomy.

The court also recommended that the mother attend a parenting course so that she could acquire the necessary skills to encourage her son's independence. Observing mother and son during the joint interview persuaded me that she could, with professional guidance, accomplish that task.

Hearing past the words

In each of the case studies cited here, a determination was achieved after an analysis of data gathered from many sources. One other factor that helps the forensic psychiatrist reach a conclusion is that intangible element we call intuition. With experience, forensic sleuths develop a "sixth sense" that allows them to deduce what is not being presented or said outright, information the adolescent might wish to hide for a variety of reasons, as the following case illustrates.

Case example #5

In one of my earliest custody cases, I interviewed Mark*, a 14-year-old who not only insisted on remaining in his mother's care but was adamantly opposed to the granting of any visitation rights to his father. When I asked the reason for his

---

* Denotes a name change.

feelings, he unleashed a tirade against his father that did not end until he declared, "I hate the man's guts!"

Without knowing why I said it, I replied, "No, I don't believe you hate him. I believe you love your father deeply but you are just angry with him right now."

There was no tangible evidence to support the statement but I intuitively felt it was true. After I uttered the words, Mark glared at me for a moment then turned away. When he lifted his head, there were tears in his eyes. "I do love him," he said, "I love him very much and I'm very upset that he won't be living with us anymore." His hostility was clearly a defense against feelings of guilt and abandonment.

My report recommended granting primary physical custody to the mother with liberal visitations for the father. I also suggested that Mark and his father undergo joint therapy to work through the son's feelings of rage, guilt, and abandonment, a conclusion that could not have been reached had I neglected to hear what lay hidden beneath Mark's words.

Conclusion

In every custody case—in addition to the due diligence of gathering data and reviewing reports—we must use our intuition and experience to uncover clues of our subject's true feelings. We must bear in mind the developmental tasks that the adolescent is confronting as well as the additional stresses that a divorce introduces, such as loyalty conflict, anger, and feelings of guilt and abandonment. We must remember that we are a stranger to this young person and that, in the absence of time that fosters trust, their innermost feelings may be kept hidden beneath their words. We must use tactical experience to collect as much data as possible and uncover as many clues as possible in order to determine what arrangement will be best for this young person's future. Only then can a forensic consultant ensure that the best interests of the adolescent have been served.

References

Ackerman, M. J. & Ackerman, M. C. (1997), Custody evaluation practices: A survey of experienced professionals (revisited). *Professional Psychol.: Res. & Pract.*, 28:137–145.

American Psychological Association, Committee on Professional Practice and Standards (COPPS) (1994), Guidelines for child custody evaluations in divorce proceedings. *American Psychologist*, 49:677–680.

Clark, B. K. (1995), Acting in the best interest of the child: Essential components of a child custody evaluation. *Family Law Quarterly*, 29:19–38.

Derdeyn, A. P. & Scott, E. (1984), Joint custody: A critical analysis and appraisal. *Amer. J. Orthopsychiat.*, 54:199–209.

Gardner, R. A. (1988), *Parental Alienation Syndrome*, 2nd ed. Cresskill, NJ: Creative Therapeutics.

Haller, L. H. (1981), Before the judge: The child-custody evaluation. *Adolescent Psychiatry*, 9:142–164.

Herman, S. P. (1997), Practice parameters for child custody evaluation. *J. Amer. Acad. Child & Adolesc. Psychiat.*, 36(Supplement):57S–68S.

Johnston, J. R. (2003), Parental alignments and rejections: An empirical study of alienation in children of divorce. *J. Amer. Acad. Psychiat. & the Law*, 31:158–170.

Kunin, C. C., Ebbeson, E. B., & Konecni, V. J. (1992), An archival study of decision-making in child custody disputes. *J. Clin. Psychol.*, 48:564–573.

Levy, A. M. (1986), Child custody determination: A proposed psychiatric methodology and its resultant case typology. *J. Psychiat. & Law*, 189–214.

Lewis, J. M. (1978), The adolescent and the healthy family. *Adolescent Psychiatry*, 6:156–170.

Lewis, J. M. (1985), The impact of adolescent children on family systems. *Adolescent Psychiatry*, 13:29–43.

Ohio Revised Code, Annotated, Section 3109.4. Accessed 1/16/06 at http://onlinedocs.andersonpublishing.com/oh/lpExt.dll?f=templates&fn=main-h.htm&cp=PORC.

Schwartzberg, A. Z. (1980), Adolescent reactions to divorce. *Adolescent Psychiatry*, 8: 379–392.

Schwartzberg, A. Z. (1981), Divorce and children and adolescents: An overview. *Adolescent Psychiatry*, 9:119–132.

Schwartzberg, A. Z. (1986), The adolescent in the remarriage family. *Adolescent Psychiatry*, 14: 259–270.

Speth, E. (1995), Factors affecting children's power to choose their caretakers in custody proceedings. *Custody Newsletter*, Issue #12/13, December 13, 1995. Available at http://www.pace411.com/newsletter12–13.html. Accessed 1/16/06.

Tooley, K. (1976), Antisocial behavior and social alienation post divorce: The "man of the house" and his mother. *Amer. J. Orthopsychiat.*, 46:33–42.

Wallerstein, J. S. & Kelly, J. B. (1996), *Surviving the Breakup: How Children and Parents Cope With Divorce.* New York: Basic Books.

Wallerstein, J. S., Lewis, J. & Blakeslee, S. (2000), *The Unexpected Legacy of Divorce: A 25 Year Landmark Study.* New York: Hyperion.

12 Talking about sexual side effects
Countering don't ask, don't tell

Ashley Harmon

Winning paper for the American Society for Adolescent Psychiatry. Award for best paper by a resident in psychiatry.

Abstract

It is indisputable that sexuality plays a significant role in adolescent development and is intertwined in much of adolescent psychopathology as well. Yet, sexuality is often left unexplored in clinical practice (Andrews, 2000). Regardless of the reasons for this—whether it is the result of the clinician's anxiety or the patient's—the understanding of the meaning of his or her sexuality is crucial to effective treatment. The purpose of this chapter is to explore the helpful role that discussions about sexuality can play in the treatment of adolescent patients and how the failure to do so may affect the patient's compliance. It will illustrate how discussions of sexuality may be explored within the context of sexual side effects that patients may experience, secondary to psychopharmacologic treatment.

Sexual activity as normal and risky behavior

From its beginning, psychoanalytic thought describes the importance of sexuality in adolescent development (Moore and Rosenthal, 1993). Nonetheless, information about normal sexual development in adolescence has remained incomplete. Numerous surveys have focused on facts and figures, but shied away from asking about subjective aspects of sexual experience (Yates, 2003). For example, the Youth Risk Behavior Surveillance System (YRBSS), sponsored by the Centers for Disease Control (CDC), monitors teenagers' sexual behavior as part of its concern about the health risks posed by adolescent sexual activity. According to data from the 2003 YRBSS, 47 percent of U. S. high school students reported ever having sexual intercourse. Nationwide, 7.4 percent of students had sexual intercourse for the first time before the age of 13 years. Approximately one third of students surveyed had had sexual intercourse in the three months preceding the survey. Of note, the percentage of sexually active students who used a condom during their last sexual intercourse increased from 46 percent in 1991 to 63 percent in 2003 (Centers of Disease Control and Prevention, 2004). From a public health perspective, sexual behavior in adolescents is considered a "risk-taking" behavior. This is indeed true when one considers the increased risk of sexually transmitted diseases and pregnancy. These data also remind us that in normal psychosexual development in contemporary North America, physical expression of sexuality precedes emotional and cognitive development regarding the meaning of sexual activity (Beausang, 2000).

The facts that sexual activity is normative for many of today's adolescents, and that such behavior carries with it significant risks, underscore the importance of discussing sexuality with teenage patients. In addition to providing opportunities for interventions to promote health and safety, such discussions can aid in the diagnostic process. An example is the determination of when sexual behavior represents the symptom of hypersexuality that is associated with psychopathology and when it represents normal development. In addition to mood states, sexual activity patterns can be indicative of sequelae from traumatic experiences (Saewyc, Magee, and Pettingell, 2004). In addition to clarifying a diagnostic picture, understanding what sexual activity means to an adolescent within the context of relationship may shed light on their interpersonal styles and abilities.

The fact that a high proportion of adolescents are sexually active also means that they are likely to have major concerns about medications that affect sexual function. Failure to anticipate these concerns may result in poor adherence to medication regimens. One way of introducing the topic of sexuality in a neutral way is to discuss sexual side effects. This should be done in the context of discussing medication in general, for reasons that will be discussed in the following section.

General issues related to medication and adolescents

There are complex psychodynamic meanings associated with having medications prescribed and taking them, as Chubinsky and Rappaport (2006) have recently discussed. They point out that meanings impact psychosocial treatment and vice versa in a complex, dynamic way. They also state that an approach that takes into account the meaning of the patient's symptoms to him or her—that is, one that incorporates a biopsychosocial framework—is imperative to making the correct diagnosis, understanding symptoms, and monitoring clinical improvement. They maintain this is true whether a psychiatrist is providing both psychotherapy and medication management or whether the treatment of a patient is split between two clinicians. They point out that a strong therapeutic alliance can facilitate a patient's sharing his or her experience of symptoms, exploring ambivalence, or agreeing to take medication.

Most would agree that building an alliance with an adolescent is critical to treatment. At the same time, such an alliance is particularly fragile with an adolescent (Meeks and Bernet, 2001). A strong therapeutic alliance facilitates treatment compliance. This is especially true when the treatment involves medications with side effects. When the side effects involve sexual functioning, they are likely to be particularly concerning in a group where there are already significant concerns about being "normal" and anxieties about sexual functioning (Robinson, 2001). Meeting with an adolescent alone and discussing the limits of confidentiality are common ways that clinicians attempt to build alliances. Exploring the psychodynamic meanings of medications to the patient impacts the alliance by helping the patient feel that the psychiatrist is interested in what is important to him or her. The importance of sexual dysfunction for adolescents is illustrated in the following case example.

Case example #1

J.J. is a 14-year-old male who presented to the outpatient clinic after being referred by his school for declining academic performance and irritability. Upon evaluation, it was determined that he was significantly impaired in several functional domains, including school, family, and peer relationships. The use of a medication was discussed, and his parents were in favor of initiating a trial of a selective serotonin reuptake inhibitor (SSRI). Individually, the psychiatrist discussed the use of medication with the patient and explored his ambivalent feelings about taking medications. Potential side effects were discussed, but sexual dysfunction was not emphasized. J.J. responded to treatment. His grades improved in school, and he became more social. After a period of months, the physician received a phone call from parents reporting that J.J. was refusing to take his medications. Upon discussing the noncompliance with the patient, sexual dysfunction was uncovered as a major contributor. J.J. reported anorgasmia during his first sexual encounters. This left him feeling embarrassed and shattered his self-esteem. He stopped the medicine after reading about it on the Internet. He did not feel that he could discuss this with the psychiatrist because he assumed that the psychiatrist would not take it seriously. It is impossible to know if discussing the potential sexual side effects at the time of initiation would have changed the course of treatment; however, the possibility that it may have is worth considering.

What we know about sexual side effects of psychotropic medications in general

Many psychotropic medications have sexual side effects, a major concern when they are prescribed for adults. Sexual side effects associated with SSRIs, as well as with the newer atypical antipsychotics, have been studied extensively in adult populations. However, the older generation of antidepressants (monoamine oxidase inhibitors and tricyclic antidepressants) and conventional antipsychotics (phenothiazines and butyrophenones) are also associated with sexual side effects (Meston and Frolich, 2000; Cutler 2003).

Rosen, Lane, and Menza (1999) critically reviewed the evidence of sexual side effects associated with SSRI use in adults. In one of the most comprehensive reviews of this topic, they concluded from available data that the incidence of sexual side effects from SSRIs varied from a small percentage to more than 80 percent. In a survey of psychiatrists, Hellewell (2000) estimated that the prevalence of sexual dysfunction, secondary to conventional antipsychotics, was 28 percent in women and 40 percent in men. However, if the patients' perceptions of a problem are surveyed, the prevalence increases to 40 percent in women and 60 percent in men (Hellewell, 2000; Cutler, 2003). This finding suggests that, in general, physicians are not attuned to this discussion of their patient's functioning.

The wide range of incidence reported in the literature further suggests the difficulty in studying sexual function, a complex phenomenon and one that many patients and clinicians are uncomfortable discussing. In addition, there are numerous methodological problems in studying sexual side effects from medications that are used to treat psychiatric illness (Scharko, 2004). Psychiatric disorders are commonly associated with a decrease in sexual desire, arousal, and function (Rosen, 1999; Piazza, Markowitz, Kocsis et al., 1997). This makes it difficult to determine when sexual dysfunction is related to the illness itself or to the medication used to treat the illness (Rosen et al., 1999; Cutler, 2003). In addition, many studies rely on spontaneous reporting of side effects—a methodology that may result in underreporting of side effects (Michelson, Bancroft, Targum, Kim, and Tepner, 2000). Only some clinical trials utilize systematic assessment of sexual functioning. Systematic methods such as direct questioning and use of reliable questionnaires and rating scales elicit a higher incidence of sexual dysfunction (Rosen et al., 1999; Michelson et al., 2000). The end result of all this variability in assessment methods is that it is difficult to compare conclusions and generalize information. Despite these difficulties, if results occur repeatedly, one can feel fairly confident they are significant, and numerous clinical trials have shown a dose-related association between SSRIs and sexual dysfunction (Montejo-Gonzalez Llorca, Izquierdo et al., 1997; Rosen et al., 1999).

Specific sexual side effects associated with psychotropics (antidepressants and antipsychotics) include ejaculatory dysfunction, decreased sexual interest (libido), decreased arousal (vaginal lubrication or erectile function), and delayed or absent orgasm (Rosen et al., 1999; Segraves, 1993; Piazza et al., 1997; Cutler 2003). These side effects are summarized in Table 12.1.

The evidence for the affect on orgasmic functioning in both men and women is strongest because of the relative ease of measuring it (Rosen et al., 1999; Cutler 2003). Additional side effects—though less common—include priapism (penile and clitoral) from SSRIs and antipsychotics (conventional and atypical). Retrograde ejaculation has long been specifically identified with thioridazine (a conventional antipsychotic), yet there have also been rare reports of this side effect with other conventional antipsychotics (Meston and Frohlich, 2000; Cutler 2003; Compton and Miller, 2001; Kotin, Wilbert, Verberg and Soldinger, 1976). The atypical antipsychotics have shown to have fewer sexual side effects than conventional agents (Cutler, 2003).

Multiple mechanisms have been proposed for medication-induced sexual dysfunction (Rosen et al., 1999). These mechanisms include various neurotransmitter systems using serotonin, dopamine, prolactin, acetylcholine, and norepinephrine (Rosen et al., 1999). The mechanism of action has been postulated to involve both

Table 12.1 Common Sexual Side Effects Reported From the Use of Antidepressants and Antipsychotics.

Drugs Studied	Reported Side Effect	Comment
SSRIs (paroxetine, fluoxestine, fluvoxamine, sertraline, citalopram)	Delayed or absent ejaculation, delayed or absent orgasm, erectile dysfunction, decreased libido	Adult and adolescent data, paroxetine worse offender than other SSRIs
TCAs (nortriptyline and clomipramine) and MAOIs	Delayed ejaculation, delayed orgasm, erectile dysfunction	Adult data
Atypical Antipsychotics (clozapine, olanzapine, ziprasidone, risperidone)	Decreased libido, transient increase in serum prolactin level, ejaculatory delay, erectile dysfunction, delay or absent orgasm	Adult data, risperidone— most substantial elevation of serum prolactin levels
Conventional Antipsychotics (haloperidol, thioridazine)	Elevated prolactin serum level, erectile dysfunction, orgasmic dysfunction, ejaculatory disturbance	Adult data, similar side effects suspected for other conventional antipsychotics, cases of retrograde ejaculation reported with thioridazine

Note: Adapted from Rosen et al. (1999), Cutler (2003), and Scharko (2004).

the central and peripheral nervous systems (Meston et al., 2000; Cutler, 2003). The SSRIs and antipsychotics elicit an effect on several of these systems directly. For example, SSRIs and the newer, atypical antipsychotics both affect serotonin and dopamine directly for their mechanism of action but also produce various levels of anticholinergic and antiadrenergic blockade as well. Serotonin acts as a neurotransmitter in the CNS and participates as part of the normal sexual-response cycle through its peripheral vasodilatory and vasoconstrictor effects (Cutler, 2003).

Prolactinemia is associated with SSRIs as well as conventional and atypical antipsychotics (Rosen et al., 1999; Cutler 2003). Serotonergic input (as occurs with SSRIs) increases the release of prolactin from the hypothalamus, as does dopaminergic blockade (Rosen et al., 1999). Elevated prolactin levels are associated with inhibition of sexual desire and erectile dysfunction (Rosen et al., 1999; Meston et al., 2000; Cutler 2003). In addition, prolactin is directly implicated in amenorrhea and galactorrhea (Cutler, 2003). Risperidone causes dose-related increases in prolactin concentrations (Cutler, 2003). Other atypical antipsychotics, including olanzapine and ziprasidone only cause transient increases in prolactin concentration whereas clozapine and quetiapine do not appear to affect prolactin (Cutler, 2003).

What we know about sexual side effects in adolescents

Increasingly, psychotropic medications are being prescribed to children and adolescents (Scharko, 2004). If information is incomplete about sexual side effects in adults, it is not surprising that it is extremely meager with regard to adolescents. To the best of my knowledge, there are only two references specifically addressing adolescent sexual side effects from psychotropic medications. One is a literature review of SSRI-induced side effects in adolescents, focusing on sexual dysfunction, and the other is a letter to the editor discussing the sexual effects of SSRIs in five patients aged 15–18 years old. Given these are the only reports in the literature, I will review and discuss them in detail.

Scharko (2004) reviewed pediatric clinical trials, clinical reviews, treatment guidelines, case reports, and MedWatch® reports to determine what the incidence of sexual dysfunction is in the adolescent population. He found that approximately one-third of the clinical reviews and treatment guidelines raised some concern about SSRI-induced sexual side effects. Only eight MedWatch® reports were filed. Of the clinical reviews, treatment guidelines, and clinical trials that mentioned sexual dysfunction, the discussions were very limited. By comparing the incidence of sexual side effects to that of more common side effects such as insomnia and dry mouth (which are comparable in adults and adolescents), he concluded that although the data are limited, the incidence of sexual side effects is likely similar in adolescents to that in adults. He recommended that sexual side effects be directly addressed in future clinical research involving adolescents to more accurately understand the significance of the problem.

In a letter to the editor, Robinson (2001) discussed the occurrence of sexual side effects in five adolescents aged 15–18 years who were treated with an SSRI in an outpatient setting. The author used patient self-reports and a lengthy questionnaire designed for adults to evaluate sexual functioning. One patient reported "improvement" of sexual functioning because of increased ejaculatory latency. Two patients reported impairment experienced impaired physical arousal that resulted in poor compliance. Two reported no change in sexual function.

Apart from the importance of eliciting information from patients about whether they are experiencing sexual side effects, discussions about the possibility of such side effects can have a salutary effect on the treatment process, whether it be psychotherapy combined with medication management, or medication management alone, as the following section will discuss.

Sexual side effects as an entrée to further discussion and treatment

Some teens are reluctant to discuss sex with a new physician for many reasons including, but not limited to, the question of confidentiality. Clinicians themselves are often anxious about bringing up the topic. Discussing sexual side effects as a prescribing physician can be helpful in curbing the clinician's anxiety about beginning the discussion about sex as well as facilitating disclosure on the part of the teenager. A nonjudgmental, fact-finding perspective can pave the way to a more thorough sexual history and show the adolescent that the clinician is open to further discussion of the subject. If the adolescent is hesitant to discuss the topic, one does not have to push. The patient knows that the physician is willing to talk about it and is interested in it. As the alliance strengthens, the patient can initiate a discussion of the topic, or the clinician can return to it. The following case illustrates how discussion of medication side effects can open a path to discussion of concerns about sexuality.

Case example #2

A.T. is a 16-year-old female who presented to the clinic for outpatient treatment, following an inpatient hospitalization for suicidal thoughts and depression. On the initial visit, the child psychiatry fellow inquired about the efficacy and tolerability of the antidepressant medication that was initiated on the inpatient unit. The patient and clinician discussed possible sexual side effects. A thorough sexual history was taken at this time. The patient began once-weekly psychotherapy and continued the medication. The overarching theme in the early therapy was her experience of the empathic failures on the part of family and friends. She felt misunderstood and isolated. During the second month of treatment, the patient began inquiring about possible sexual side effects. In the course of the discussion that ensued, she described a sexual encounter that she had experienced several years earlier, which had left her feeling ashamed and vulnerable. Together she and the clinician processed what the sexual encounter meant to her. In subsequent sessions, she continued to present questions about sex and the feelings associated with it.

Within this process, topics related to sexual safety, such as contraceptives and sexually transmitted diseases, were discussed. Most importantly, the patient was able to describe a previous sexual encounter that occurred years earlier where she was forced to engage in acts she was unsure of. Although the patient had not reported this trauma at the initial evaluation, despite having been asked about it, the openness of the clinician to discuss sexual side effects probably allowed the patient to mention the trauma at a later time.

This case illustrates how discussing sexual side effects with patients may set a tone of openness in the therapy. A nonjudgmental stance on the part of the therapist allows the patient to ask questions that might otherwise go unasked (Andrews, 2000). The ensuing discussion can impact physical health—by educating about safe sex—as well as psychological health. In this particular case, the patient was able to work through a traumatic experience.

Conclusion

In summary, many psychotropic medications prescribed carry the potential for sexual side effects, and the mechanisms for these are complex, involving many neurotransmitter systems. Adolescent sexual activity may be a manifestation of psychopathology, or may represent normal psychosexual development. Understanding an adolescent's sexual concerns and development is part of a comprehensive psychiatric evaluation. As prescribing psychiatrists, we should consider it imperative to discuss and understand sexual side effects from our patients' perspectives. They are relevant to the diagnostic and treatment processes, providing crucial information about excessive risk-taking behavior, traumatic experiences, and interpersonal relationships. But this crucial aspect of the assessment is often inadequately addressed, especially when the psychiatrist is not the therapist. The practice of integrated, dual-treatment, ongoing psychosocial and biological intervention from the same clinician is becoming more of a rarity than standard practice. Initiating a discussion about the sexual side effects of medications offers a helpful entrée into this challenging topic. Discussing sexual side effects can lead to improved compliance, facilitate open discussion, and lead to opportunistic interventions to reduce risk and promote healthy development. Little has been written about medication-induced sexual side effects in adolescents, and even less about the long-term effects. Given that adolescents are still undergoing sexual development, not knowing the long-term effects should give us pause. In addition to the improvement in monitoring and reporting of sexual side effects in adolescents, continuing research should focus on how psychotropic medications may effect normal biological and psychosocial development.

References

Andrews, W. (2000), Approaches to taking a sexual history. *J. Women's Health & Gender-Based Med.*, 9 Suppl 1:S21–4.

Beausang, C. (2000), Personal stories of growing up sexually. *Issues in Comprehensive Pediatric Nursing*, 23:175–192.

Centers of Disease Control and Prevention. *Surveillance Summaries*, May 21, 2004. MMWR 2004: 53 (no. SS–2).

Chubinsky, P. & Rappaport, N. (2006), Medication and the fragile alliance: The complex meaning of psychotropic medication to children, adolescents, and their families. *J. Infant, Child, Adolesc. Psychother.* 5:111–123.

Compton, M. & Miller, A. (2001), Priapism associated with conventional and atypical antipsychotic medications: A review. *J. Clin. Psychiat.*, 62:362–366.

Cutler, A. (2003), Sexual dysfunction and antipsychotic treatment. *Psychoneuroendocrinology*, 28:69–82.

Hellewell, J. (2000), Tolerability of patient satisfaction as determinants of treatment choice in schizophrenia: A multi-national survey of the attitudes and perceptions of psychiatrists towards novel and conventional antipsychotics (poster). Presented at the 13th European College of Neuropsychopharmacology Congress, Munich, Germany.

Kotin, J., Wibert, D., Verberg, D., & Soldinger, S. M. (1976), Thioridazine and sexual dysfunction. *Amer. J. Psychiat.*, 133:82–85.

Meeks, J. & Barnet, W. (2001), *The Fragile Alliance*. Malabar, FL: Krieger Publishing.

Meston, C. & Frohlich, P. (2000), The neurobiology of sexual function. *Arch. Gen. Psychiat.*, 57:1012–1030.

Michelson, D., Bancroft, J., Targum, S., Kim, Y., & Tepner, R. (2000), Female sexual dysfunction associated with antidepressant administration: A randomized, placebo-controlled study of pharmacologic intervention. *Amer. J. Psychiat.*, 157:239–243.

Montejo-Gonzalez, A., Llorca, G., Izquierdo, J. A., Ledesma, A., Bousono, M., Calcedo, A., Carrasco, J. L., Ciudad, J., Daniel, E., De la Gandara, J., Derecho, J., Franco, M., Gomez, M. J., Macias, J. A., Martin, T., Perez, V., Sanchez, J. M., Sanchez, S., & Vicens, E. (1997), SSRI-induced sexual dysfunction: Fluoxetine, paroxetine, sertraline, and fluvoxamine in a prospective, multicenter, and descriptive clinical study of 344 patients. *J. Sex Marital Ther.*, 23:176–94.

Moore, S. & Rosenthal, D. (1993), *Sexuality in Adolescence*. New York: Routledge.

Piazza, L., Markowitz, J., Kocsis, J. H., Leon, A. C., Portera, L., Miller, N. L., & Adler, D. (1997), Sexual functioning in chronically depressed patients treated with SSRI antidepressants: A pilot study. *Amer. J. Psychiat.*, 154:1757–1759.

Robinson, M. (2001), Antidepressant-induced sexual dysfunction in adolescents. *Can. J. Psychiat.*, 46:185.

Rosen, R., Lane, R., & Menza, M. (1999), Effects of SSRIs on sexual function: A critical review. *J. Clin. Psychopharmacol.*, 19:67–85.

Saewyc, E., Magee, L., & Pettingell, S. (2004), Teenage pregnancy and associated risk behaviors among sexually abused adolescents. *Perspectives on Sexual and Reproductive Health*, 36:98–105.

Scharko, A. (2004), Selective serotonin reuptake inhibitor-induced sexual dysfunction in adolescents: A review. *J. Amer. Acad. Child Adolesc. Psychiat.*, 43:1071–1079.

Segraves, R. (1993), Treatment-emergent sexual dysfunction in affective disorder: A review and management strategies. *J. Clin. Psychiat. Monogr.*, 11:57–60.

Yates, A. (2003), Normal sexual development. In *Textbook of Adolescent Psychiatry*, ed. R. Rosner. London, England: Arnold Publishing Co., pp. 85–92.

Section III

When clinical skills are not enough

Psychiatric enigmas

13 Reactive attachment disorder in adolescence

John P. Kemph and Kytja K. S. Voeller

Abstract

Reactive attachment disorder (RAD) has received increasing attention as a possible explanation of severe behavioral disturbances in children and adolescents. Its etiology is hypothesized as related to failure of attachment beginning in infancy. Although the diagnosis of reactive attachment disorder (RAD) is usually made in early childhood, the diagnosis may be carried over into adolescence. In some cases, the diagnosis may be made for the first time in adolescence if there is sufficient information in the history to make the diagnosis retrospectively. It is unlikely that the diagnosis of RAD can be made in the absence of comorbid diagnoses in adolescence because these children usually have symptoms which meet the criteria for other diagnoses, such as attention deficit disorder (ADHD), post-traumatic stress disorder (PTSD), oppositional defiant disorder (ODD), mood disorder, or conduct disorder (CD) by the time they become early or mid-adolescent ages. During development, additional diagnostic criteria for other DSM-IV diagnoses may be observed. Although a comorbid diagnosis of ADHD, ODD, and/or CD might appear to take precedence over RAD, with the burgeoning information in genetics it may be useful to know that RAD was present or may still be present in the symptom complex of an individual patient. This chapter presents an overview of the issues involved in nosology and possible etiology, with particular emphasis on neurobiology and genetics. Case vignettes are used to illustrate the challenges to treatment that these patients present.

Definition and diagnosis

The diagnostic criteria for RAD are primarily "a markedly disturbed and developmentally inappropriate social relatedness, in most contexts beginning before 5 years" of age, which is associated with pathogenic care (American Psychiatric Association, 2000, p. 130). Two types of RAD are described: (1) inhibited and (2) disinhibited. In the literature on RAD there are many descriptions and definitions. It seems appropriate, although possibly oversimplified, to state that the basic problem is a disturbance in the child-parent relationship, i.e., in social relatedness.

The disturbance in social relatedness continues to be the defining feature of the disorder, despite evolution of the diagnostic criteria. Diagnostic criteria for RAD have changed across various editions of the Diagnostic and Statistical Manual of

Mental Disorders of the American Psychiatric Association. For decades "attachment" was synonymous with the infant–caregiver relationship. Subsequently, the diagnosis of RAD has come to apply to the child's appearing to have a disturbance in social relatedness to others. The term "reactive" is used in the sense that the condition is considered to be a reaction to "pathogenic care," which is defined as characterized by "persistent disregard for the child's basic emotional needs for comfort, stimulation and affection." It is sometimes also associated with "a prolonged disregard for the child's physical needs" (American Psychiatric Association, 2000, p. 130). The constellation of behavioral and physical signs seen in infants with RAD include lack of a smiling response and lack of an auditory alerting response with head-turning towards the caregiver's voice, coupled with abnormal physical development such as failure to thrive with no apparent physical cause.

Changes in successive editions of the DSM reflected a broadening of the diagnostic criteria and the age groups to which RAD could be applied. In DSM-III (American Psychiatric Association, 1980) the diagnosis basically applied to infants aged 8 months or less and, therefore, was limited in its application to older children. In the DSM-III-R (American Psychiatric Association, 1987) the age of onset was extended up to less than 5 years of age. Also, instead of a detailed list of symptoms, the criteria consisted of the presence of either of two patterns of social relatedness: (1) excessively inhibited, ambivalent interactions with others, and (2) indiscriminate social behaviors. A history of "grossly pathogenic care" was still a required criterion. DSM-IV (American Psychiatric Association, 1994) employed a more detailed description which took into consideration research findings which indicated that individual children respond in different ways to pathogenic care. Some may form selective attachments, while others may develop RAD in situations in which the care is not "grossly pathogenic." Therefore, the term "grossly" was eliminated from the DSM-IV description of diagnostic criteria. There was no change in the RAD diagnostic criteria in DSM-IV-TR (American Psychiatric Association, 2000), and the two subtypes designated "inhibited" and "disinhibited" remained.

Contributions from attachment research

Early investigators observed infants who had been neglected, abused, or both, and developed hypotheses to account for the profound disturbances in development they saw. Spitz (1946) called the condition he observed "anaclitic depression in infants." Bowlby (1982) considered the disorder a reaction to attachment and loss. Provence and Lipton (1962) made further observations on infants in institutions. Ainsworth, studying attachment in normal children, developed the "strange situation" procedure which assessed the child's response to a change involving the caretaker (1978). In the strange situation, the baby is exposed to two brief separations from its mother and a brief exposure to a stranger. Ainsworth observed "coherent" and "incoherent" patterns of response to this stressful situation. Infants with "coherent" responses fell into three subtypes: "secure type" infants communicated interactively with their mothers and were able to use the mother as a secure base for exploration. The other two coherent subtypes were described as "insecure avoidant" and "insecure resistant." Infants manifesting an "incoherent response" showed evidence of disorganized attachment, defined as freezing, appearing fearful in the presence of the mother, engaging in stereotypy and "contradictory behavior." Subsequent research has shown that attachment patterns formed in infancy tend to be stable over time, even into adulthood (Waters et al., 2000), although they are subject to change in response to the vicissitudes of development. The relationship between various types of attachment and psychopathology is complex, and empirical research in this area is still in its early stages. Disorganized attachment has been associated with aggression and disruptive behavior later in development (Lyons-Ruth, 1996) and with dissociative symptoms (Ogawa, Stroufe, Weinfield, Carlson and Egeland, 1997). While youngsters who do not have attachment disorders are likely to be securely attached, those who have disorganized attachments do not necessarily develop attachment disorders (Boris et al., 2004).

There have been few studies on the reliability of RAD diagnoses. Using their own diagnostic criteria, which differ slightly from those of the DSM, researchers in infant psychiatry have been able to demonstrate that attachment disorders can be reliably diagnosed in high-risk samples of young children (Boris et al., 2004).

Overlap with other disorders

RAD can be confused with other disorders. Some children with disturbances in social relatedness have communication problems that can be classified as a language disorder. Presumably the longer the child is deprived of normal language stimulation, the more severe the communication problem becomes. Richters and Volkmar (1994) suggest that, when communication problems are present, the diagnosis should be considered one of atypical development rather than a disorder of attachment, per se.

Children with RAD may become disruptive and disorganized with poor affect regulation and poor frustration tolerance, as well as inattention, impulsivity, and hyperactivity. By the time these children reach adolescence, they have often accumulated numerous comorbid diagnoses such as ADHD, and/or ODD, and/or CD, and/or PTSD. Also, one of the several mood-disorder diagnoses may be associated with RAD.

The following two case vignettes are examples of adolescents with RAD.

Case #1

A 14-year-old girl was brought, by her adoptive parents, to an outpatient psychiatric clinic because of their concern about recent changes in her behavior. She had been adopted at 7 years of age by a middle-aged couple after their own children had grown up. This couple felt that they were ready to accept the challenge of raising a problem child. This child had been neglected and abused by her natural parents, and she had behaved aggressively and destructively in several foster homes. Initially these adoptive parents had taken this child into their home as a foster child. They had been given the history of her previous pathogenic care and difficult behavior and her diagnosis of RAD. They were instructed to provide a warm and loving environment, as this was considered her greatest need at that time. The couple was successful in providing a supportive environment in spite of the child's testing the limits of their patience periodically, and they proceeded to adopt her. After the reassurance provided by the adoption, the relationship between the child and parents continued to improve until some typical adolescent peer interactions occurred. Several other girls in her school, with whom she had become acquainted, formed a clique and rejected her. At the same time, because she had blossomed into an attractive young girl, boys showed her increased attention. Eventually she started dating the boys and became sexually promiscuous. These behaviors prompted her parents to seek help at an outpatient clinic, where they were provided with counseling from a social worker and medical care for the girl from a psychiatrist. She was given the comorbid diagnoses of RAD, ADHD, ODD, and mood disorder, not otherwise specified. The parents were supported in their attempts to set limits on these behaviors, and the child was given therapy that was aimed to improve self esteem and impulse control. She was also given several trials of psychotropic medicines. The therapeutic program provided by the clinic and the parental intervention were not successful in controlling her sexual acting out. She became more oppositional and refused to see both her therapist and her psychiatrist. Her behaviors became more dangerous to her health. She ultimately appeared to have some of the characteristics of borderline personality disorder and eventually was placed in a residential program for adolescents with borderline personality disorder.

Case #2

A 15-year-old girl was referred by the school because of symptoms of truancy and refusal to cooperate. Both the patient and the mother agreed that the mother had neglected her children. Her father had deserted the family when the patient was an infant. Her mother suffered from severe recurrent major depressive episodes during which she was unable to care for her children. The mother refused therapy. Although the patient was in an outpatient treatment program, she continued to refuse to attend school. She was admitted to an adolescent unit in a psychiatric hospital for an intensive evaluation which included an inpatient behavioral assessment, a complete psychiatric and psychological workup, and a neurological assessment. Her admitting diagnoses were RAD and ODD. The results of the intensive evaluation indicated that she had never developed an attachment to her mother (RAD) and later had never developed any deep investment in her peers. Her reality testing was usually good, but occasionally she became very unrealistic and her judgment was often poor. She was angry and depressed much of the time in the hospital and she was given the diagnosis of borderline personality disorder. The neurologist who consulted on the case had some concern that she might have evidence of prefrontal executive function deficits, which have been reported to be associated with borderline personality disorder (Zelkowitz, Paris, Guzder et al., 2001).

In both of these cases, the adolescents had received pathogenic care as infants and, in subsequent developmental years, they did not form relationships with either adults or peers that might foster attachment. In the first case, the opportunity for attachment was there—her adoptive parents had provided loving care—but the child had been unable to incorporate the investment that the parents had provided. She was not able to form the identification necessary to internalize those characteristics that are needed to accept parental guidance. She was unable to reciprocate, either showing appreciation for the parental effort, or by attempting to meet some of the parental expectations.

In the second case, the diagnosis of RAD was made retrospectively during outpatient care by a child psychiatrist and was substantiated in the course of an intensive inpatient evaluation and treatment effort. During treatment, both patients demonstrated projective identification in which they projected a transferred identity on the therapist. In the opinion of the staff, this provided them with a justification for their inability to form an emotionally close relationship.

Etiological factors in RAD

Longitudinal studies on the impact of early deprivation

Longitudinal studies on brain function, cognition, and social behaviors of children, raised under conditions of extreme deprivation, have also provided further information about the impact of severe early deprivation on later development (Chisholm, 1998; Chugani, Behen, Muzik, et al., 2001; Kaler and Freeman, 1994; Rutter, Anderson-Wood, Beckett, et al., 1999). The unfortunate "experiment of nature" in Romanian orphanages has provided a rich source of data about the response of infants to defective maternal care. As infants, children in these orphanages were exposed to severe deprivation—some for as long as 42 months—and were then adopted and raised by families in the U.K. They have been extensively studied longitudinally by Rutter and colleagues, and many publications appeared on their findings. The highly pathogenic nature of this environment has been well documented. There is a linear relationship between the intensity of care (that is, the caretaker to child ratio), the duration of deprivation, and the child's subsequent behavior. Low intensity of care and prolonged duration of exposure to social deprivation were found to be associated with higher levels of disturbed attachment, delays in physical growth and cognitive development, and later psychopathology

(Chisholm, 1998; O'Connor and Rutter, 2000; Smyke, Dumitrescu, and Zeanah, 2002; Ellis, Fisher, and Zaharie, 2004). At age 6 years, some of these children manifested normal social and cognitive development, whereas others did not (Rutter and O'Connor, 2004). This finding suggests that some children are constitutionally more vulnerable than others to early pathogenic environments and that their pathological behaviors may persist, despite later nurturing environments and treatments. Thus, although early pathogenic care is an important factor, it is not the only one. The interaction between the child, the caregiver, and the child's developmental trajectory depends on a number of factors, particularly the child's resilience and ability to respond to later appropriate care.

Disruption of normal brain development by intrauterine or perinatal encephalopathic factors (e.g., maternal illness, exposure to drugs and toxins, prematurity, hypoxia, or malnutrition) is likely to increase the negative impact of environmental factors on later development and the infant's ability to respond to its caretaker. This is particularly true when the neural systems that underlie social relatedness and autonomic function are affected. Infants who are extremely irritable and inconsolable, on one hand, or those who are lethargic and unresponsive, on the other, pose a formidable challenge to even the most caring and experienced mother. In some infants, the neural network underlying social-emotional behaviors may be impaired to the extent that the infants cannot develop appropriate attachment, even in the most optimal situation (Pipp-Siegel, Siegel, and Dean, 1999).

A second, obviously important factor involves the mother's ability to relate to and nurture the infant. Poor mothering appears to be, at least in part, the result of the mother's own early experience, as well as being the result of cognitive, emotional, and environmental factors (Wilson, Kuebli, and Hughes, 2005). There are relatively few studies about the effect of poor mothering on a mother's own behavior, but there is a large research literature indicating that nonhuman primate mothers who were abused as infants have a high likelihood of being abusive to their own children. This is observed in infants raised by their biological as well as nonbiological abusive mothers (Maestripieri, 2005). Another factor is the mother's emotional state and ability to regulate her own behavior in response to the child, particularly if the child is hard to manage. In one large longitudinal study, maternal anxiety during pregnancy and postpartum maternal depression constituted independent and additive risks for emotional and behavioral problems in the child at age 4 years. This was true even after controlling for factors such as maternal smoking, alcohol use, the child's birth weight relative to gestational age, maternal age, gender, and socioeconomic status (O'Connor, Heron, and Glover, 2002).

There is also the matter of "goodness of fit" in the mother-child dyad. Mothers who cannot adapt their interactive styles to a quiet, relatively unresponsive infant or to one who is irritable and demanding will also enhance the child's risk of developing RAD. The more the mother is able to provide external regulation of the infant's level of arousal, the less likely the environment will be a pathogenic trigger.

However, even in this highly pathogenic situation there is some variability in the child's response. Somatic growth appears to be one factor that has a bearing on the child's response to deprivation in an institutional setting. Although growth retardation occurs in most of these children (the mean stature of the children in Romanian orphanages fell 1.6 standard deviations below the mean), there is a difference in the behavior of large and small children. In the study reported by Ellis, Fisher, and Zaharie (2004), smaller children manifested more anxiety/affective symptoms, whereas large physical size was associated with higher levels of disruptive behavior and aggression. The authors speculated that, in an institutional setting, aggression might be adaptive because the more aggressive the behavior, the more likely the child would receive both food and attention.

Mechanisms by which deprivation of care may alter brain function

Early deprivation of maternal care results in a series of somatic, emotional, and neurocognitive sequelae, which reflects a complex interplay between environmental input and brain development. A prominent aspect of the impact on brain function, with significant downstream effects on emotional regulation, is the dysfunction of the hypothalamic–pituitary–adrenal (HPA) axis that occurs in RAD. This dysfunction is characterized by elevated cortisol release in response to stressful events. Adults who experienced childhood abuse and neglect manifest hyperreactivity of the hypothalamic-pituitary-adrenal (HPA) axis and autonomic nervous system in response to stress, compared to adults who did not have this history. This effect is particularly striking in women who are also depressed (Heim et al., 2002). These observations in adults are echoed in the finding that children, who spent over eight months of their first year of life in a Romanian orphanage, had daytime cortisol levels that were significantly higher than controls. The longer they remained in the orphanage, the higher the levels (Gunnar, Morison, Chisholm, and Schuder, 2001).

In response to stress, corticotrophin release factor (CRF) is secreted by the hypothalamus, stimulating the release of ACTH from the pituitary, which in turn stimulates the release of cortisol from the adrenals. CRF is regulated through negative feedback by glucocorticoid receptors which are located in the hippocampus as well as several other areas of the brain. Thus, highly sensitive glucocorticoid receptors will down-regulate CRF. Of particular interest, given the role of serotonin in depression and hippocampal function, is the fact that serotonin increases the expression of hippocampal glucocorticoid receptor expression as well as expression of nerve-growth-factor-inducible factor A (*NGFI-A*) gene. This gene is a member of the family of zinc-finger transcription factors encoded by immediate-early genes, and induced by a wide variety of extra cellular stimuli. *NGFI* is involved in cell proliferation, synaptic activation, and long-term potentiation, and is distributed in several brain regions, including the hippocampus. This aspect of RAD has been the focus of considerable preclinical research and is likely to be of considerable importance to the clinician.

To explain these persisting effects of maternal deprivation on the HPA axis, Meaney and Szyf (2005) have proposed an intriguing theory which ties the impact of poor maternal care to experience-dependent chromatin plasticity. In other words, experience in the neonatal period results in long-lasting changes in the system regulating CRF in response to stress. The experimental animal model involved the newborn rat. (However, similar effects of early maternal deprivation have also been demonstrated in male rhesus monkeys: see Winslow, 2005.) Adult rats raised by mother rats that are devoted lickers-and-groomers showed reduced ACTH and corticosterone responses to acute stress, in comparison to rats raised by less attentive rat mothers (Liu et al., 1997). Good maternal care is associated with a significant increase in hippocampal glucocorticoid receptor messenger RNA and protein expression, as a result of increased binding *NGFI-A* to the glucocorticoid receptor, which results in increased sensitivity of hippocampal glucocorticoid receptors and results in the down-regulation of CRF. This effect appears to be directly related to the effect of early maternal care, as switching rat pups born to low-intensity lickers and groomers to mothers who are intense lickers and groomers results in more stress-resistant adult rats. (Reversing this switch also has the opposite effect.) The mechanism involves the demethylation of the *NGFI-A* gene. Immediately after birth, the *NGFI-A* gene is methylated and therefore silenced. Intense licking and grooming activates serotonin receptor–7 (5-HT$_7$ receptor), which in turn demethylates *NGFI-A*, and increases *NGFI-A* transcription. The resulting increased sensitivity to CRF by the hippocampal glucocorticoid receptor down-regulates cortisol secretion. Meaney and Szyf (2005) note that since DNA methyltransferases and demethylases are present in neurons and repetitive stimulation can alter the methylation status of neuronal genes, this is a more general model explaining how early environmental impacts can alter the brain's genetic programming.

This theory is particularly exciting because it integrates the clinical data which demonstrates the marked hyperreactivity of the HPA axis in response to stress in individuals who suffered neglect and abuse in early childhood. It also provides a model that explains how early experience affects genetic programming, and in turn results in persistent patterns of brain function which become "organic" (Kemph, 1964). Moreover, although these effects remain through life if not treated, there are manipulations in the laboratory setting that can reverse the genetic effects. The theory also suggests a number of approaches to therapy as it may be possible to demethylate some genes that have been silenced.

The infant's genetic constitution

There are other components of the way poor maternal care affects the infant. Infants are born with different genetic profiles, and recent clinical and animal studies have provided strong evidence that the infant's genetic make-up is an important factor in the response to pathogenic environments. Genes that regulate the neuronal systems which underlie the infant's ability to relate to its mother and the infant's resilience in the face of adversity will affect response to pathogenic rearing conditions. It is likely that some infants are genetically more susceptible to develop disturbed attachment. Genes involving the dopaminergic, vasopressin, serotoninergic, and μ-opoid systems have been implicated.

Dopaminergic system   Dopamine is involved in social relatedness through the mesolimbic system. Mesolimbic dopamine plays an important role in motivation, attention, and response to rewards. At this point it is not clear whether dopamine may be involved in the hedonic aspect of social bonding or in enhancing the relevance of social signals (Insel, 2003). However, in one study young adults who were exposed to poor maternal care and did not bond well with their mothers displayed a significant increase in ventral striatal dopamine release (as well as cortisol) in response to a stressor (Pruessner, Champagne, Mesney, et al. 2004). This, as well as other studies, would suggest that poor maternal care affects the dopaminergic system (Liu et al., 1997).

The dopamine D4 receptor (DRD4) has a number of polymorphisms which are related to effective dopaminergic signaling. One polymorphism involves a 48-base pair-variable number of tandem repeats in exon III. The number of repeats is associated with differential sensitivity to dopamine. Thrill-seeking, novelty-seeking (Benjamin, Patterson, Greenberg, Murphy, et al. 1996), drug addiction, (Kotler et al., 1997), and impulsive/compulsive behavior (Comings et al., 1999) in various adult populations around the world have been linked to the DRD4 gene polymorphisms. There are numerous studies reporting an association of the dopamine receptor D4 gene with ADHD, but these associations have certainly not been universally replicated in all samples and in all ethnic populations.

Some studies have reported that behavior in infancy is influenced by various DRD4 polymorphisms. In a sample of 122 Italian infants, those infants with the long DRD4 receptor polymorphism scored more poorly on adaptability, in contrast to those with the short allele. At five months of age these differences were no longer observed (De Luca, Rizziardi, Buccino, et al., 2001). However, at 3 years of age, toddlers with a long DRD4 7-repeat allele were more reactive than those who were homozygous for the short DRD4 (4/4) alleles. No relationship to adaptability, extraversion, or exploratory behaviors was noted (De Luca et al., 2003).

Lakatos and colleagues (2002) described a study on a cohort of 12- to 13-month-old infants that employed Ainsworth's strange situation paradigm described above (Ainsworth et al, 1985). They noted that 71 percent of the infants with a pattern of disorganized behavior in the strange situation had at least one 7-repeat DRD4 allele, compared to 29 percent of children who did not manifest this type of disorganized response.

In a subsequent study by the same group, it was found that when the 7-repeat DRD4 allele as well as a C → T substitution in the 5'-promoter region of the DRD4 gene (resulting in reduced transcriptional efficiency) (Okuyama et al., 2000) were present, the odds ratio for disorganized behavior increased tenfold (Lakatos et al., 2002). Gervai, Nemoda, Lakatos et al. (2005) have subsequently replicated this finding and noted that the *absence* of the 7-repeat haplotypes and the C → T substitution in the promoter region enhanced optimal development of early attachment. However, these findings have not been replicated in all populations (Bakermans-Kranenburg & Van Ijzendoom, 2004).

It would be simplistic to assume that the infant's genetic constitution is the only factor in this equation. However, a given genotype may increase an infant's vulnerability to a pathogenic environment. Support for this notion comes from a 14-year longitudinal study of Finnish children followed into adulthood. Keltikangas-Jarvinen and colleagues, (2004) noted that when the parents were strict disciplinarians, had little tolerance for the normal activity of young children, and were emotionally remote, the offspring who had 2- or 5-repeat alleles of the DRD4 gene were much more likely to manifest the novelty-seeking profile (above the 10th percentile compared to Finnish norms) than those who did not have those alleles. In a more accepting child-rearing environment, the DRD4 genotype did not appear to have an effect.

Moreover, it is also likely that it is not just one set of genes but rather the interaction of multiple genes that contributes to the infant's response to its environment. There is a complex relationship between serotonin and dopamine. Auerbach and colleagues (2001) reported that 12-month old infants with the DRD4 7-repeat allele manifested a higher level of activity in a free play situation and were less interested in structured block play and had greater difficulty sustaining attention to a task than infants who did not have the 7-repeat allele. They also examined the relation of the serotonin transporter promoter (5-HTTLPR) gene in this situation and noted that infants with two short 5-HTTLPR alleles appeared less fearful when approached by a stranger and were also less involved in the structured block play. They also noted a significant interaction between DRD4 7-repeat allele and the serotonin transporter promoter (5-HTTLPR) gene in relation to sustained attention.

Monoamine Oxidase-A (MAO-A)   Monoamine oxidase-A is one of the enzymes involved in the metabolism of monoamine neurotransmitters. A variable number tandem repeat polymorphism at the promoter of the *MAO-A* gene (mapped to Xp11.23–11.4) results in enhanced enzymatic activity and, thus, would be expected to moderate increased catecholamine levels, which occur in response to pathogenic care. Testing the hypothesis that enhanced *MAO-A* activity would result in less psychiatric pathology in children raised in pathogenic environments, Caspi et al., (2002) observed, in a large longitudinal study, that boys raised in pathogenic environments who had a genotype conferring high levels of *MAO–A* expression were less likely to develop antisocial problems. Of the sample, only 12 percent of the males had the low-activity *MAO–A* genotype combined with early maltreatment. However, 85 percent of them developed some form of antisocial behavior and they accounted for 44 percent of the cohort's violent convictions.

The Vasopression System Arginine vasopressin has also been shown to play an important role in social behaviors, including affiliation and attachment, via the arginine vasopressin receptor 1A, by mediating the relationship between social stimuli and brain reward circuits (Winslow and Insel, 2002; Insel, 2003). The arginine-vasopressin (AVP) system also plays an important role in linking social signals to the mesocorticolimbic circuit. The AVP receptor 1A gene (AVPR1A) has been identified as an autism-susceptibility gene (Wassink, Piven, Vieland et al., 2004). Male monkeys with social deficits also show reduced binding of AVP to limbic structures. CRF binding is reduced in these monkeys as well (Winslow, 2005).

The μ-Opioid System This system plays a critical role in the development of positive affective states linked to the mother. Since social contact provides opioid-mediated comfort, and social separation typically causes distress similar to opiate withdrawal (Panksepp, Sivily and Normansell, 1985), mouse pups lacking the μ-opioid gene would not experience either state because of the absence of the receptors which regulate the responses to social isolation or comfort. This is supported by studies on μ-opioid "knockout" mouse pups (those in whom the gene has been inactivated). In contrast to normal pups, those lacking the μ-opioid gene do not emit distress signals when removed from their mothers, although they do express distress in the presence of other cues (Moles, Kieffer & DÁmato, 2004). The implication of these findings is that infants with atypical μ-opioid genetic profiles might tolerate absence of a mother figure to a greater extent than those with intact μ-opioid systems.

The Serotonergic System This system is also likely to be involved in the way children respond to abuse and neglect. As noted above, serotonin plays a crucial role in the hippocampal NGFI-A/glucocortical receptor transcription. There is a large literature on the relationship of serotonin to mood, social anxiety, and obsessive-compulsive behaviors, and both age and gender appear to be important variables in this relationship. There are two common polymorphisms in a variable repeat sequence of the serotonin transporter promoter (5-HTT—also known as SLC6A4) gene (on chromosome 17q11.1-q12). The long variant has more than twice the activity of the short variant, which is associated with reduced transcription and lower transporter activity. A number of studies have described an association between one or two copies of the short allele of the 5-HTT promoter polymorphism and depression and suicidality in response to stressful life events (Caspi et al., 2003) although this has not been replicated in all populations (Gillespie, Whitfield, Williams, et al. 2005). The short 5-HTT promoter polymorphism has also been associated with increased activation of the amygdala and increased fear and anxiety-related behaviors (Hariri, Mathay, Tessitore et al., 2002). Children with one or two copies of the short allele manifested higher levels of shyness and behavioral inhibition (antecedents of social anxiety disorder). There are also differences in patterns of cortical activation in these children in response to angry and neutral faces (Battaglia, Ogliari, Zanoni et al., 2005).

Implications for treatment

The previous section provides a neurobiological explanation for the mechanisms by which environmental factors program patterns of brain function, and in turn set up long-lasting behaviors. Once a pattern of behavior is established over a long period of time in a human being at any age, it is embedded in the genetic patterns that regulate neuronal activity, and in turn lead to behavioral patterns and identity (Kemph, 1964). The longer the pattern exists the more difficult it is to change, but change should nonetheless still be possible. A rational approach to treatment in these cases would likely involve both pharmacologic as well as persistent behavioral interventions. In addition to generating new nerve cells in the hippocampus, enhancing the development of new patterns of neuronal connectivity should encourage the development of more adaptive ideas and behavior patterns to replace old patterns.

With appropriate care, in our experience, some children with RAD show remarkable improvement. For example, an adopted 6-year-old boy with typical autistic behavior improved over the course of a year with once-a-week therapy for the boy and counseling for the adoptive parents, and with the supportive environment of his new family. After one year he was able to function in a regular classroom and interact well with his adoptive family. Although the developmental history was not available, this child had probably not been genuinely autistic, but rather was "quasi-autistic" as suggested by Rutter et al. (1999).

Another case is that of a 15-year-old boy who was treated in a children's psychiatric hospital for more than a year. Although he initially appeared to be only minimally responsive to this intensive treatment, he subsequently showed evidence of having benefited from it through having made an attachment to the therapist. This boy had a stormy history of failure to form an attachment to his mother, other adults, peers, or therapists. He had frequent rages and dangerous behavior directed toward peers and adults, including therapists. He was considered to have RAD and conduct disorder. Although some progress was made in forming an attachment to his therapist in the hospital (they met for daily therapy sessions for one year), his behavior did not improve to the point that it could be tolerated. The episode that triggered his transfer occurred when, in a rage, he had produced eight knives that he had obtained, and twirled in a dangerous fashion, attempting to cut the staff. He was eventually talked into going into the quiet room with his therapist, where he relinquished the knives and quickly settled down when he realized he had gone too far. Shortly thereafter he was transferred to a high-security state hospital. Eventually, after discharge from that hospital, he returned for a visit with his former therapist at the children's psychiatric hospital. He told his former therapist that while he was alone in the secure hospital he began to recall many of the discussions he had had with his therapist, and began to determine what he had to do to work his way out of the hospital. He stated that he now realized that the work with his former therapist was helpful. Apparently he had internalized enough of the relationship with his former therapist, possibly through identification, for him to use to his advantage in the state hospital.

The management of RAD children, whether by parents or therapists, requires considerable patience with very little expectation of immediate success. These children and adolescents are often aggressive and oppositional, frequently testing the limits of external controls or rules. Their caretakers must be prepared to forego any expression of appreciation from these patients for the caretaker's efforts; they must be prepared for frequent negative testing behavior. Some people are more capable of providing this type of care than others. When these patients become aggressive and oppositional it is often helpful to wait briefly and patiently before giving any response, allowing time for the patient to become more aware of the situation which he/she is creating and then help the patient to respond more appropriately. Many repetitions will be necessary to promote the development of new, more adaptive behaviors (which in turn involves "resetting" some of the underlying neuronal pathways and, by altering transcription patterns—possibly by some of the mechanisms described above—changing some of the underlying genetic programs). The older the patient the more time and repetitions will be required. Optimistically, the younger the patient the better the chance of getting results relatively soon. Caretakers and the therapists must be capable of providing care even with negative response or little reward from patients initially, and even after many repetitions there will be only minimal reward. If we consider the biological processes that must occur in order to achieve a change in behavior, we may be less impatient with the intractable quality of the behaviors.

We earlier discussed the importance of "goodness of fit" in fostering attachment. Goodness of fit has been cited as helpful in planning which caretakers would be a good fit for which patients. Colin (1996) has noted that clinicians should be aware of the importance of goodness of fit between the child and the adoptive parent and how well they function together in their relationship. A change in that relationship, if needed, may require prolonged intensive treatment with the child and the caregiver. To demonstrate the goodness of fit, two brief case vignettes will be described. Both cases were being treated by the same child psychiatrist who provided psychotropic medicines for the child and brief counseling for the mother and child. Both of these children had been given the comorbid diagnoses of RAD, ADHD, ODD, and PTSD. One was a 10-year-old adopted girl who had previously been placed in several foster homes. The adoptive mother needed occasional reassuring responses from the child that would indicate that she was trying to become part of the family, but the child gave much more negative than positive feedback. The girl was very oppositional and the mother responded with disappointment or anger. The mother frequently requested help, in the form of increased medication, which provided only partial improvement in behavior. The mother was often in tears and became increasingly desperate and tired. Eventually she gave up custody of the child to social services.

The other child was an 11-year-old girl who had been adopted at 4 1/2 years of age from a Russian orphanage. The mother said that the first two years were horrible, with no professional support. She brought the child to an outpatient clinic when the child was 7 years old. Over time, and with the help of the therapist, the adoptive mother became very capable of managing the child's oppositional behavior. In the psychiatrist's office at the clinic, when the child became aggressively oppositional, the mother would wait, briefly allowing the child to think about what she had done, and pleasantly, usually with a smile, teach the child how to respond more appropriately.

A much better result was obtained in the second of these two examples, which illustrate different expectations and reactions to the child on the part of the adoptive parent. In the second case, the adoptive mother was more realistic in her expectations. She was not seeking personal gratification from her interventions with the child and was not reacting immediately or intensely in a negative way to the child's behavior. There are obviously many issues involved in the treatment of these children, but, considering the potential reactivity of these children to stressors, the lack of heightened negative emotional responses from the caretakers may be an important factor.

Because of the extreme difficulties these children present for caregivers, not to mention social agencies and therapists who deal with them, various outpatient and inpatient programs have appeared in the United States specializing in treating patients with RAD. The examples described by Wilson (2001) utilize stimulation therapy, parental counseling, psychiatric consultation, and "holding therapy." Control via coercive techniques is heavily emphasized in some of these programs. According to Wilson, holding therapy attempts to recreate the bonding cycle that an infant may have experienced with a parent by the following procedure: the therapist holds the child's head in his/her lap to maintain eye contact while others restrain the arms and the legs. The therapist confronts the child with questions such as "Who has control now?" and "I know you hate, but who ends up suffering?" Thirty hours in 10 days is devoted to this procedure. Wilson concludes, given the complexity of the factors underlying the development of RAD, and the fact that there are no peer-reviewed outcome studies, "until such time as holding techniques can be empirically validated to improve the condition of RAD without excessive stress to the child, parents may be well advised to consider other options in the treatment of a child with RAD" (Wilson, 2001, p. 49). Holding therapy and an even more extreme form of restraint and noxious stimulation known as "rebirthing therapy" are quite controversial and have been condemned by the American Psychiatric Association (2002), which stated, "there is no scientific evidence to support the effectiveness of such interventions," and cited "a strong clinical consensus that coercive therapies are contraindicated in this disorder." The American Academy of Child and Adolescent Psychiatry (AACAP) has issued a similar statement (2003), noting that at least six documented child fatalities have occurred related to the use of these methods. The AACAP also notes "these techniques also violate the fundamental human rights of the children subjected to them. The AACAP therefore urges that these coercive, dangerous and ineffective practices be discontinued." Nonetheless, these techniques continue to have their supporters, and persist in some programs as a treatment in both outpatient and inpatient settings.

As noted previously, some children raised in pathogenic environments develop symptoms resembling borderline personality disorder. These patients often manifest prefrontal executive dysfunction (Zelkowitz et al., 2001). Further support for frontal dysfunction is supported by the finding of hypometabolism in orbitofrontal cortex on positron emission tomography scans (Soloff et al., 2003). These observations are consistent with the disruption of dopaminergic transmission observed following exposure to maternal deprivation (Liu et al., 1997; Preussner et al., 2004). If these symptoms develop in adolescence the APA guidelines for treatment of patients with borderline personality disorder (American Psychiatric Association, 2001) may be helpful in therapy.

Although children and adolescents with RAD may improve in cognitive function, language, and motor development, changes in social relatedness may be more difficult to achieve. The following is a brief example of improved social relatedness in an adolescent:

A 13 ½-year-old boy had been adopted by his great aunt when he was 10 years old. When the boy was just 8 months of age, the aunt was surprised to learn that her niece had an infant son about whom she had never heard. When the aunt visited the child she was appalled at the poor physical condition of this tiny infant. The mother told her aunt that she had been on several illicit drugs while she was pregnant with this child. She was addicted to several drugs, including methamphetamine and cocaine, and had not cared for the child properly. The infant's great aunt tried repeatedly to get her niece to give the child to her and let her take the child into her home. Her own children had been raised well and were out of the home. Finally, when the child was 10 years old, the mother of the child allowed her aunt to adopt him. At that time the aunt took the child to a children's psychiatric clinic where he was diagnosed as having ADHD, ODD, and, by history, RAD. The child and caretaker were seen in counseling by a social worker and by a psychiatrist who provided medicine. During three years of treatment as an outpatient, the patient developed an attachment to his adoptive mother and his oppositional and aggressive behavior were largely diminished. However, he continued to give a negative initial response to most questions, albeit with a pleasant demeanor. Then he would use his adoptive mother's knowledge and support to formulate a plan for further responses, reminiscent of the infant using its attachment to its caretaker when a secure attachment has been established. He made friends among peers and the adoptive mother's grownup children. When a new child psychiatrist interviewed the dyad the adoptive mother was asked if there was any mental illness in the family, the boy said immediately, "My mom." The adoptive mother then explained that his mother had been diagnosed as having schizophrenia in addition to substance abuse. Although this boy lags behind academically and has symptoms of inattentiveness and distractibility, which require medication, he has formed a secure attachment to his adoptive mother during puberty and early adolescence and this provides a basis for trust and for him to further his development in the future.

Effective pharmacotherapy

The fact that various genetic features appear to play a role in RAD, as we have discussed above, suggests that carefully conceptualized approaches to medication might be helpful. When more information is available about a specific child's genotype, particularly as it relates to neurotransmitters and drug metabolism, this should provide a rational approach, utilizing pharmacogenomic information, to managing some of the behaviors that characterize RAD. However, even in the absence of such information, systematically targeting the oxytytocin, μ-opiod, serotonin, and dopaminergic systems may be helpful in combination with persistent behavioral interventions.

Summary

Although the examples of patients with RAD described in this article are anecdotal and not conclusive proof that some adolescents with RAD can develop an attachment when this has not occurred at a younger age, they offer the possibility that such behavioral changes may occur in an appropriate setting. The recent advances in knowledge of genetics and neuroscience are reassuring, because there is evidence that brain function and some of the genetic factors underlying brain-function structure can be modified to allow for changes in behavior.

RAD is a useful diagnosis for some adolescents who present with "markedly disturbed and inappropriate social relatedness in most contexts," when the problem in relatedness can be demonstrated to have begun in early childhood and there is a history of "pathogenic care," or at least profound disturbance in the parent-child relationship. RAD places children at risk for other psychopathology as they grow older, so that by the time a child with RAD becomes an adolescent other diagnoses have been added, such as ADHD, ODD, PTSD, mood disorder, or CD. When a diagnosis of RAD is first made during childhood, it may be carried over into adolescence. A diagnosis of RAD may be made in older children or adolescents retrospectively from history. Although the DSM criteria associate RAD with pathogenic care, research in infant psychiatry has led to a revision of thinking about this disorder, positing that the nature of the parent-child relationship may be critical. Irritability or uncontrolled negative-affective responses on one end of the spectrum, as well as indifferent, apathetic responses on the other— on the part of *either* the parent or the child — may interfere with the development of normal attachment, particularly if there is a "poor fit." The caretaker's ability to regulate the infant's arousal level may be one important factor. Another factor may involve the influence of different genotypes which will determine, in part, the sensitivity of the child to the pathogenic situation. Treatment of RAD requires many repetitions of appropriate thoughts and behaviors over a prolonged period of time to foster the changes necessary to form new neuronal patterns, which may enable the adolescent to develop socially acceptable relationships with other people. Skillful use of medication may also be helpful.

References

Ainsworth, M. D. S., Blehar, M. S., Waters, E. & Wall, S. (1978), *Patterns of Attachment.* Hillsdale, NJ: Erlbaum.

_____ (1985), *Patterns of Attachment: A Psychological Study of the Strange Situation.* Hillsdale, NJ: Erlbaum.

American Academy of Child and Adolescent Psychiatry (2003), Policy Statement on Coercive Interventions for Reactive Attachment Disorder. Washington, DC, Author. 12–5–1910. Available at http://www.aacap.org/publications/policy/ps48.htm. Accessed 10/12/05.

American Psychiatric Association (1980), *Diagnostic and Statistical Manual of Mental Disorders,* 3rd ed. Washington, DC: American Psychiatric Association.

_____ (1987), *Diagnostic and Statistical Manual of Mental Disorders,* 3rd ed., *Revised.* Washington, DC: American Psychiatric Association.

_____ (1994), *Diagnostic and Statistical Manual of Mental Disorders,* 4th ed. Washington, DC: American Psychiatric Association.

_____ (2000), *Diagnostic and Statistical Manual of Mental Disorders,* 4th ed., text revision. Washington, DC: American Psychiatric Association.

American Psychiatric Association (2001), Practice guideline for the treatment of patients with borderline personality disorder. *Amer. J. Psychiat.,* 158 (Suppl. 10):1–52.

American Psychiatric Association (2002), Reactive Attachment Disorder Position Statement. Washington, DC, American Psychiatric Association. Available at http://www.psych.org/edu/other_res/lib_archives/archives/200205.pdf. Accessed 10/12/05.

Auerbach, J. G., Faroy, M., Ebstein, R., Kahana, M., & Levine, J. (2001), The association of the dopamine D4 receptor gene (DRD4) and the serotonin transporter promoter gene (5-HTTLPR) with temperament in 12-month-old infants. *J. Child. Psychol. Psychiat.,* 42:777–783.

Bakermans-Kranenburg, M. J. & Van Ijzendoorn, M. H. (2004), No association of the dopamine D4 receptor (DRD4) and −521 C/T promoter polymorphisms with infant attachment disorganization. *Attach. Hum. Dev.,* 6:211–218.

Battaglia, M., Ogliari, A., Zanoni, A., Citterio, A., Pozzoli, U., Giorda, R., Maffei, C., & Marino, C. (2005), Influence of the serotonin transporter promoter gene and shyness on children's cerebral responses to facial expressions. *Arch. Gen. Psychiat.,* 62:85–94.

Benjamin, J., Li, L., Patterson, C., Greenberg, B. D., Murphy, D. L., & Hamer, D. H. (1996), Population and familial association between the D4 dopamine receptor gene and measures of novelty seeking. *Nature Genet.,* 12:81–84.

Boris, N. W., Hinshaw-Fuselier, S. S., Smyke, A. T., Scheeringa, M. S., Heller, S. S., & Zeanah, C. H. (2004), Comparing criteria for attachment disorders: Reliability and validity in high risk samples. *J. Amer. Acad. Child & Adolesc. Psychiat.,* 43:568–577.

Bowlby, J. (1982), *Attachment and Loss,* vols. 1–3, 2nd ed. New York: Basic Books.

Caspi, A., McClay, J., Moffitt, T. E., Mill, J., Martin, J., Craig, I. W., Taylor, A., & Poulton, R. (2002), Role of genotype in the cycle of violence in maltreated children. *Science,* 297:851–854.

Caspi, A, Sugden, K., Moffitt, T. E., Taylor, A., Craig, I. W., Harrington, H., McClay, J., Mill, J., Martin, J., Braithwaite, & A., Poulton, R. (2003), Influence of life stress on depression: Moderation by a polymorphism in the 5-HTT gene. *Science,* 301:386–389.

Chisholm, K. (1998), A three year follow-up of attachment and indiscriminate friendliness in children adopted from Romanian orphanages. *Child Dev.* 69:1092–1106.

Colin, V. (1996), *Human Attachment.* New York: McGraw Hill.

Chotai, J., Serretti, A., Lattuada, E., Lorenzi, C., & Lilli, R. (2003), Gene environment interaction in psychiatric disorders as indicated by season of birth variations in tryptophan hydroxylase, serotonin transporter and dopamine receptor (DRD4) gene polymorphisms. *Psychiatry Res.,* 119:99–111.

Chugani, H. T., Behen, M. E. Muzik, O. Juhasz, C. Nagy, F., & Chugani, D. C. (2001), Local brain functional activity following early deprivation: A study of postinstitutionalized Romanian orphans. *Neuroimage,* 14:1290–1301.

Comings, D. E., Gonzalez, N., Wu, S., Gade, R., Muhleman, D., Saucier, G., Johnson, P., Verde, R., Rosenthal, R. J., Lesieur, H. R., Rugle, L. J., Miller & W. B., & MacMurray, J. P. (1999), Studies of the 48 bp repeat polymorphism of the DRD4 gene in impulsive, compulsive, addictive behaviors: Tourette syndrome, ADHD, pathological gambling, and substance abuse. *Amer. J. Med. Genet.,* 88:358–368.

DeLuca, A., Rizzardi, M., Buccino, A., Alessandroni, R., Salvioli, G. P., Filligrasso, N., Novelli, G., & Dallapiccolo, B. (2003), Association of dopamine D4 receptor (DRD4) exon III polymorphism with temperament in 3-year-old infants. *Neurogenetics,* 4:207–212.

DeLuca, A., Rizzardi, M., Torrente, I. Alessandroni, R., Salvioli, G. P., Filligrasso, N., Dallapiccolo, B., & Novelli, G. (2001), Dopamine D4 receptor (DRD4) polymorphism and adaptability trait during infancy: A longitudinal study in 1- to 5-month-old neonates. *Neurogenetics,* 3:79–82.

Ebstein, R. P., Novick, O., Umansky, R., Priel, B., Osher, Y., Blaine, D., Bennett, E. R., Nemanov, L., Katz, M., & Belmaker, R. H. (1996), Dopamine D4 receptor (D4DR) exon III polymorphism associated with the human personality trait of novelty seeking. *Nature Genet.* 12:78–80.

Gervai, J., Nemoda Z., Lakatos, K., Ronai, Z., Toth, I., Ney, K., & Sasvari-Szekely, M. (2005), Transmission disequilibrium tests confirm the link between DRD4 gene polymorphism and infant attachment. *Amer. J. Med. Genet. B Neuropsychiatr. Genet.,* 132:126–130.

Gillespie, N. A., Whitfield, J. B., Williams, B., Heath, A. C., & Martin, N. G. (2005), The relationship between stressful life events, the serotonin transporter (5-HTTLPR) genotype and major depression. *Psychol. Med.,* 35:101–111.

Gunnar, M. R., Morison S. J., Chisholm, K., & Schuder, M. (2001), Salivary cortisol levels in children adopted from Romanian orphanages. *Dev. Psychopathol.,* 13:611–628.

Hariri, A. R., Mattay, V. S., Tessitore, A., Kolachana, B., Fera, F., Goldman, D., Egan, M. F., & Weinberger, D. R (2002), Serotonin transporter genetic variation and the response of the human amygdala. *Science,* 297:400–403.

Heim, C., Newport D. J., Heit S., Graham, Y. P., Wilcox, M., Bonsall, R., Miller, A. H., & Nemeroff, C. B. (2000), Pituitary-adrenal and autonomic responses to stress in women after sexual and physical abuse in childhood. *J. Amer. Med. Assn.,* 284:592–597.

Insel, T. R. (2003), Is social attachment an addictive disorder? *Physiol. Behav.,* 79:351–357.

Kaler, S. R. & Freeman B. J. (1994), Analysis of environmental deprivation: cognitive and social development in Romanian orphans. *J. Child Psychol. Psychiat.,* 35:769–81.

Keltikangas-Jarvinen, L., Elovainio M., Kivimaki M., Lichtermann, D., Ekelund, J., & Peltonen, L. (2003), Association between the type 4 dopamine receptor gene polymorphism and novelty seeking. *Psychosom. Med.,* 65:471–476.

_____, Raikkonen, K., Ekelund, J., & Peltonen, L. (2004), Nature and nurture in novelty seeking. *Mol. Psychiat.,* 9:308–311.

Kemph, J. P. (1964), The symptom or character trait may become "organic." *Amer. J. Psychiat.,* 120:1085-1088.

Kotler, M., Cohen, H., Segman, R., Gritsenko, I., Nemanov, L., Lerer, B., Kramer, I. Zer-Zion, M., Kletz, I., & Ebstein, R. P. (1997), Excess dopamine D4 receptor (D4DR) exon III seven repeat allele in opioid-dependent subjects. *Mol. Psychiat.*, 2:251–254.

Kotler, M., Manor I., Sever Y., Eisenberg, J., Cohen, H., Ebstein, R. P., & Tyano, S L. (2000), Failure to replicate an excess of the long dopamine D4 exon III repeat polymorphism in ADHD in a family-based study. *Amer. J. Med. Genet.*, 96:278–281.

Lakatos, K., Nemoda, Z., Toth, I. Ronai, Z., Ney, K., Sasvari-Szekely, M., & Gervai, J. (2002), Further evidence for the role of the dopamine D4 receptor (DRD4) gene in attachment disorganization: Interaction of the exon III 48-bp repeat and the –521 C/T promoter polymorphisms. *Mol. Psychiat.*, 7:27–31.

_____, Toth, I., Nemoda, Z., Ney, K., Sasvari-Szekely, M., & Gervai, J. (2000), Dopamine (D4) receptor (DRD4) gene polymorphism is associated with attachment disorganization in infants. *Mol. Psychiat.*, 5:633–637.

Liu, D., Diorio J., Tannenbaum B., Caldji, C., Francis, D., Freedman, A., Sharma, S., Pearson, D., Plotsky, P. M., & Meaney, M. J. (1997), Maternal care, hippocampal glucocoticoid receptors, and hypothalamic-pituitary-adrenal responses to stress. *Science*, 277:1659–1662.

Lyons-Ruth, K. (1996), Attachment relationships among children with aggressive behavior problems: The role of disorganized early attachment patterns. *J. Consult. Clin. Psychol.*, 64:64–73.

Maestripieri, D. (2005), Early experience affects the intergenerational transmission of infant abuse in rhesus monkeys. *Proc. Natl. Acad. Sci. USA*, 102:9726–9729.

Mattick, J. S. (2003), Challenging the dogma: The hidden layer of non-protein-coding RNAs in complex organisms. *BioEssays*, 25:930–939.

Meaney, M. J. & Szyf, M. (2005), Maternal care as a model for experience-dependent chromatin plasticity? *Trends Neurosci.*, 28:456–463.

Moles, A., Kieffer, B. L., & D'Amato, F. R. (2004), Deficit in attachment behavior in mice lacking the mu-opioid receptor gene. *Science*, 304:1983–1986.

O'Connor, T. G., Ben-Shlomo, Y., Heron, J., Golding, J., Adams, D., & Glover, V. (2005), Prenatal anxiety predicts individual differences in cortisol in pre-adolescent children. *Biol. Psychiat.*, 58:211–217.

O'Connor, T. G., Heron, J., & Glover, V. (2002), Antenatal anxiety predicts child behavioral/emotional problems independently of postnatal depression. *J. Amer. Acad. Child Adolesc. Psychiat.*, 41:1470–1477.

O'Connor, T. G. & Rutter, M. (2000), The English and Romanian adoptees (ERA) study team. Attachment disorder behavior following early severe deprivation: Extension and longitudinal follow-up. *J. Amer. Acad. Child Adolesc. Psychiat.*, 39:703–712.

Ogawa, J. R., Stroufe, L. A., Weinfield, N. S., Carlson, E. A., & Egeland, B. (1997), Development and the fragmented self: Longitudinal study of dissociative symptomatology in a nonclinical sample. *Dev. Psychopathol.*, 9:855–879.

Okuyama, Y., Ishiguro, H., Nankai, M., Shibuya, H., Watanabe, A., & Arinami, T. (2000), Identification of a polymorphism in the promoter region of DRD4 associated with the human novelty seeking personality trait. *Mol. Psychiat.*, 5:64–69.

Panksepp, J., Sivily, S. M., & Normansell, L. A. (1985), Brain opioids and social emotions. In: *The Psychobiology of Attachment and Separation*, ed M. Reite & T. Field. New York: Academic Press, pp. 33–49.

Pipp-Siegel, S., Siegel, C., & Dean, J. (1999), Neurological aspects of the disorganized/disoriented attachment classification system: Differentiating quality of the attachment relationship from neurological impairment. In: *Atypical Attachment in Infancy and Early Childhood Among Children at Developmental Risk. Monograph of the Society for Research in Child Development*, ed. J. I. Vondra & D. Barnett. 64:25–44.

Provence, S. & Lipton, R. (1962), *Infants in Institutions*. New York: International Universities Press.

Pruessner, J. C., Champagne, F., Meaney, M. J., & Dagher, A. (2004), Dopamine release in response to a psychological stress in humans and its relationship to early life maternal care: A positron emission tomography study using [11C]raclopride. *J. Neurosci.* 24:2825–2831.

Richters, M. M. & Volkmar, F. R. (1994), Reactive attachment disorder in infancy and early childhood. *J. Amer. Acad. Child Adolesc. Psychiat.*, 33:328–332.

Rutter, M., Anderson-Wood, L., Beckett, C., Bredenkamp, D., Castle, J., Groothues, C., Kreppner, J., Keaveney, L., Lord, C., & O'Connor, T. G. (1999), Quasi-autistic patterns following severe early privation. *J. Child Psychol. Psychiat.*, 40:537–549.

Rutter, M. & O'Connor. T. G. (2004), Are there biological programming effects for psychological development? Findings from a study of Romanian adoptees. *Dev. Psychol.*, 40:81–94.

Rutter, M. L., Kreppner, J. M., & O'Connor T. G. (2001), Specificity and heterogeneity in children's responses to profound institutional privation. *Brit. J. Psychiat.*, 179:97–103.

Soloff, P. H, Meltzer, C. C., Becker, C., Greer, P. J., Kelly, T. M., & Constantine, D., (2003), Impulsivity and prefrontal hypometabolism in borderline personality disorder. *Psychiat. Res.*, 123:153–163.

Spitz, R. (1946), Anaclitic depression. *Psychoanalytic Study of the Child* 2:313–342. New Haven, CT: Yale University Press.

Wassink, T. H., Piven, J., Vieland, V. J., Pietila, J., Goedken, R. J., Folstein, S. E., & Sheffield, V. (2004), Examination of AVPR1a as an autism susceptibility gene. *Mol. Psychiat.*, 9:968–972.

Wilson, S. L. (2001), Attachment disorders: Review and current status. *J. Psychol.*, 135:37–51.

Wilson, S. L., Kuebli, J. E., & Hughes, H. M. (2005), Patterns of maternal behavior among neglectful families: Implications for research and intervention. *Child Abuse Negl.* 29:985–1001.

Winslow, J. T. (2005), Neuropeptides and non-human primate social deficits associated with pathogenic rearing experience. *Int. J. Dev. Neurosci.* 23:245–251.

Winslow, J. T. & Insel, T. R. (2002), The social deficit of the oxytocin knockout mouse. *Neuropeptides,* 36:221–229.

Zelkowitz, P., Paris, J., Guzder, J., & Feldman, R. (2001), Diatheses and stressors in borderline pathology of childhood: The role of neuropsychological risk and trauma. *J. Amer. Acad. Child Adolesc. Psychiat.*, 40:100–105.

14 When Clozapine doesn't work

Two case reports of treatment-refractory adolescent schizophrenia

Atara S. Stahl, Theodore Shapiro,
Margaret E. Hertzig, Wendy Turchin

Abstract

Because of the oftentimes more severe and chronic nature of schizophrenia with onset during adolescence, management of adolescents with this disorder poses an even greater challenge than it does for adults with schizophrenia. As there are very few controlled drug trials in this population, there is a significant lack of consensus in the management of adolescents with schizophrenia. This ambiguity becomes especially pronounced when physicians are faced with the difficult situation of managing an adolescent patient who appears to be refractory to treatment. Since the advent of atypical neuroleptics, accepted practice has been to treat refractory schizophrenia with clozapine. However, management of refractory schizophrenia that is resistant even to clozapine represents yet another challenge to our treatment protocols. Here we present two case reports of previously high-functioning adolescents who were diagnosed with schizophrenia and were found to be refractory to a variety of treatments, including trials of high-dose clozapine.

Introduction

Schizophrenia with onset during adolescence is a relatively uncommon disorder with follow-up that suggests devastating outcomes (Hafner and Nowotny, 1995). Because of the oftentimes more severe and chronic nature of earlier-onset schizophrenia, management of adolescents with schizophrenia poses an even greater challenge than it does for adults with this illness.

There are few controlled drug trials in this population, in part due to the relative rarity of the illness and in part due to ethical considerations of conducting drug trials with children (Clark and Lewis, 1998). As a result, there is a significant lack of consensus in the pharmacological management of schizophrenia with onset in adolescence. This ambiguity becomes especially pronounced when physicians are faced with the difficult situation of managing an adolescent patient who appears to be refractory to treatment. Since the advent of atypical neuroleptics, accepted practice has been to treat refractory schizophrenia with clozapine. However, management of refractory schizophrenia that is resistant even to clozapine represents yet another challenge to our treatment protocols. We present two case reports of previously high-functioning adolescents who were admitted to the Payne Whitney Child and Adolescent Inpatient Unit for treatment of schizophrenia. Our experience with both patients was that they were refractory to a variety of treatments, including trials of high-dose clozapine maintained for periods of over four months. Both patients became treatment dilemmas for us as they demonstrated refractoriness to what is usually considered the gold standard and "last attempt" medication option for treatment-resistant schizophrenia. To the best of our knowledge, this is the first published description of such cases. Following the case presentation, we will provide a critical review of the literature concerning treatment-refractoriness and schizophrenia with onset during childhood or adolescence.

Case examples

Case example #1

M.C. was a 17-year-old white male, admitted to the child and adolescent inpatient unit with a psychotic illness. M.C. had been "very social" and a "perfectionistic" straight-A senior at a prestigious public high school until about four months prior to admission, when his grades began falling. Around the same time, he abruptly stopped attending sessions with the outpatient psychiatrist whom he had seen weekly for several years (for vague anxiety symptoms, with no medications given). He also inexplicably missed his scholastic aptitude (SAT) exam and began "behaving bizarrely" by sleeping every day after school, avoiding his friends, constantly discussing fears that he was gay and expressing a desire to go to a Catholic university although he was raised Jewish. He became increasingly paranoid and guarded, often saying that he was "not safe at home." He was brought to the hospital psychiatric emergency room by police after he threatened to leave home in the middle of the night on New Year's Eve. The only family history available to us was that his paternal grandmother had undergone electroconvulsive treatment (ECT) for unknown reasons. He had a normal birth history, normal developmental milestones, and no significant past medical history.

M.C. was admitted with a working diagnosis of schizophreniform disorder. He was extremely guarded with poor eye contact and a marked latency in his responses to questions. He demonstrated a general paucity of content in his responses and at times was disorganized in his speech. When asked about hallucinations, thought insertion, thought withdrawal, or ideas of reference, he answered "I don't want to talk about that." Physical and neurological examinations were normal. Drug screen for cannabinoids, cocaine, opioids, and benzodiazepines was negative.

Treatment was started with olanzapine 5 mg. b.i.d. and lorazepam 1 mg. at bedtime. M.C. continued to exhibit psychotic behavior by walking around the unit naked, licking the floor, drinking his own urine, and repeatedly stating, "The FBI is following me." Haloperidol was added to the regimen three days later, and increased to a maximum dose of 6 mg. daily over the next 4 weeks, with little improvement in his psychotic behavior. After four weeks, because of his failure to respond to the medications, ECT was suggested. After the first ECT treatment, a partial response was noted, but it was not sustained. After a series of 10 ECT treatments over the course of one month, M.C. demonstrated increased spontaneity of speech and was noted to be more socially engaged than before, but his insight was judged as "poor," and he remained largely paranoid and delusional.

At this point, a decision was made to stop ECT and to initiate clozapine. Haloperidol was discontinued because of emerging Parkinsonian symptoms. Over the course of six weeks, clozapine was increased to a dose of 450 mg. daily. Throughout this trial, M.C. exhibited increased social withdrawal, impoverished thought, and inattention to grooming. Four and one-half months after admission, M.C was discharged on clozapine 450 mg. daily.

M.C. was followed in our outpatient clinic for one month following his discharge from the inpatient unit and maintained on clozapine 450 mg. daily. Over the course of the month, his functioning declined further. His negative symptoms increased, with blunted and reserved affect, marked apathy, lack of spontaneity, and impoverished thought. He continued to exhibit bizarre behavior, such as sitting naked in the dark and expressing paranoid thoughts to his mother.

At this time, M.C. was readmitted to the child and adolescent inpatient unit in the setting of a missed dose of clozapine and emerging bizarre behavior such as avoiding TVs and mirrors and walking around naked. He was started on atenolol, and his clozapine dose was increased to 600 mg. daily. During this hospitalization, he engaged in odd behavior including clapping, counting, rituals, and continued paranoid thoughts. M.C. was also socially isolated and disheveled with poor hygiene and grooming throughout the hospitalization. He was, however, able to pass a standardized state academic exam during the hospitalization. He was discharged on clozapine 600 mg. daily after one month of hospitalization.

For the subsequent 32 months, M.C. was followed in our outpatient clinic. Throughout this time, he continued the clozapine trial (maximum dose of 675 mg daily), and completed additional trials of haloperidol, methylphenidate, fluoxetine, and sertraline. Over this period of time, negative symptoms prevailed. He often missed therapy groups, sat in sessions with his eyes closed, and demonstrated significant amotivation and social isolation. His positive symptoms included moving his hands in the air to "see the shadows" and then weeping upon seeing these shadows. He continued to endorse paranoid ideation and demonstrate grossly disorganized thought. At our last point of contact with M.C., over four years after his first presentation to our facility, he remained paranoid, psychotic, and socially withdrawn. His current diagnosis is chronic paranoid schizophrenia, which has been virtually refractory to a variety of treatments including clozapine.

Case example #2

E.H. was a 17-year-old white male admitted to the child and adolescent inpatient unit for diagnostic workup of psychotic features consistent with schizophrenia. E.H. had been "well-adjusted" and had received good grades in his yeshiva class until he was about 12 years old, when he became much more socially withdrawn and began having difficulty with his schoolwork. Around this time he also became increasingly inappropriate and disruptive by assuming bizarre gestures in public, laughing inappropriately, and refusing to go to sleep until he was reassured for hours that he hadn't done anything wrong. He seemed to "live inside his imagination" and barely communicated with others.

Because E.H.'s parents did not wish to hospitalize him initially, he was treated by several different outpatient psychiatrists and given a multitude of diagnoses between the ages of 12 and 17. Throughout this five-year period, he failed trials of fluoxetine, sertraline, venlafaxine, citalopram, clomipramine, aripiprazole, divalproex, lamotrigine, risperidone, quetiapine, and olanzapine, in addition to various combinations of these medications. Much of this time, E.H. was being treated with a working diagnosis of mood disorder not otherwise specified. He showed brief periods of improved function at the beginning of each of these trials, but this improvement was always followed by a rapid decline. During the five years he was followed, he exhibited increasingly bizarre behavior and became progressively socially dysfunctional.

This patient's birth and development history were normal. He had no significant past medical history, and there is no known family history of psychiatric illness.

At the time of admission, his parents reported that E.H. had not been in school for about a year because of "lack of ability to function within the community or communicate effectively." His parents brought him to the hospital because they felt that he had not improved with any of the medication trials over the previous five years and they hoped to find a medication that "worked" by finally admitting E.H. to the hospital. On admission, E.H. was generally expressionless and had poor eye contact. He glanced about the room frequently, appeared to be responding to internal stimuli, and refused to answer questions. He seemed preoccupied and whispered in Yiddish that he "just wants peace of mind."

E.H. was started on a trial of aripiprazole 30 mg daily (as this was a relatively new agent at the time which showed promise in the literature) augmented with olanzapine 5 mg b.i.d. for two weeks, after which aripiprazole was continued alone for an additional week. Throughout the trial of aripiprazole with olanzapine, E.H. remained withdrawn, guarded, incoherent, thought blocked, and preoccupied with internal stimuli. At this point, all medications were tapered and a clozapine trial was started. He was titrated to clozapine 600 mg. daily over a three-month course, the last of which was augmented with valproic acid 1250 mg. daily. Throughout this trial, E.H. again showed no significant improvement in symptoms and was ultimately discharged with symptoms that were virtually identical to those he presented with upon admission approximately 130 days earlier.

Discussion

Schizophrenia with onset in childhood or adolescence

Since the introduction of the DSM-III in 1980, the diagnosis of schizophrenia in children and adolescents (generally referred to as early-onset schizophrenia, or EOS) has been made according to the same criteria as in adults. Research since this time has validated the similarity between EOS and adult schizophrenia and therefore has supported this decision (American Academy of Child and Adolescent Psychiatry, 2001). Neuropsychologic and neurobiologic studies generally support continuity of schizophrenia with onset in childhood and adolescence with adult-onset schizophrenia (Jacobsen and Rapoport, 1998; Kumra, Shaw, Merka, et al., 2001). Because of the similarities between EOS and adult schizophrenia, and due to the scarcity of available literature focusing on EOS, data based on schizophrenia in adults are often extrapolated to apply to schizophrenia in children and adolescents.

However, it has been noted that certain essential differences do exist between EOS and adult schizophrenia. It is fairly well-accepted that schizophrenia with onset in childhood or adolescence tends to be more severe than its adult counterpart (Kravariti, Morris, Rabe-Hesketh, et al. 2002). Hafner and Nowotny (1995) found that onset of schizophrenia before age 21 was associated with greater social impairment than was later-onset schizophrenia. Remschmidt, Schultz, Martin, et al. (1994) conclude that schizophrenic psychoses with early manifestation have a poor prognosis. Yang, Liu, Chiang, et al. (1995) suggest that onset of schizophrenia before age 15 is associated with more negative symptoms in later life. These findings support clinical observations that adolescent-onset schizophrenia may be more insidious, more chronic, and have a less favorable outcome than adult-onset schizophrenia.

While prevalence of schizophrenia in the adult population has been estimated to be about 1 percent (Meltzer, Lee, and Ranjan, 1994), reliable epidemiological data on incidence and prevalence of schizophrenia in children and adolescents are limited. It has been suggested in recent literature that about 20 percent of adult schizophrenics experience onset of their illness before age 20 (Hafner and Nawatny, 1995; Kumra, Shaw, et al. 2001). Other estimates suggest that as many as one-third of patients with schizophrenia present in childhood or adolescence (Loranger, 1984; Beratis, Gabriel, and Hoidas, 1994).

Overall, current research estimates suggest that one fifth to one third of all patients with schizophrenia are resistant to drug treatment (Conley and Kelly, 2001). Although existing data have often been too limited to make definite conclusions, many adolescents with schizophrenia do not respond or respond only partially to neuroleptics (Quintana and Keshavan, 1995). Some authors claim that children and adolescents are more prone than adults to side effects of neuroleptic treatment, and have higher rates of nonresponse (Hafner and Nowatny, 1995). Although it is uncertain whether children and adolescents with schizophrenia are actually less responsive to neuroleptic agents than are adults, earlier age of onset is reported to be a predictor of poor therapeutic response in adults (Kumra, Jacobsen, Lenane et al., 1998). Therefore, it is hardly surprising that rates of treatment refractoriness in EOS tend to be higher than those in adult-onset schizophrenia.

Approaches to pharmacologic treatment of schizophrenia in adolescents

Although the use of neuroleptics in the treatment of schizophrenia in children or adolescents has been studied in a number of trials during the past two decades, conclusions have not been definitive, and further study is warranted. Literature on treatment of refractory adolescent schizophrenia is especially limited. For example, while guidelines and protocol recommendations on the management of childhood and adolescent schizophrenia do exist, these protocols do not address management of refractory childhood and adolescent schizophrenia.

According to the practice guidelines set forth by the Practice Parameters for the Assessment and Treatment of Children and Adolescents with Schizophrenia (American Academy of Child and Adolescent Psychiatry, 2001), after a comprehensive assessment of the child or adolescent with schizophrenia, a trial of first-line antipsychotics should be initiated. First-line agents for the treatment of the psychotic symptoms associated with schizophrenia in adolescents include typical and atypical antipsychotic agents. The accepted next step, once a patient is determined to be treatment-refractory to at least two other antipsychotic drugs, including one atypical antipsychotic, is to initiate a trial of clozapine, provided the patient can tolerate it.

Further research comparing atypical antipsychotics to typical antipsychotics, and to each other, is still needed. However, current literature does show some convincing data that both typical and atypical agents can be effective in the treatment of schizophrenia occurring in children and adolescents. In several studies, typical neuroleptics have been shown to be superior to placebo in treatment of children and adolescents with schizophrenia. Pool, Bloom, Mielke, et al. (1976) compared haloperidol, loxapine, and placebo in 75 hospitalized adolescents with acute schizophrenia, using a double-blind, randomized study format over a four-week period. Investigators found significant changes from baseline regarding all treatment groups according to the Brief Psychiatric Rating Scale (BPRS) (Overall and Gorham, 1962) and Clinical Global Impressions Scale (CGI) (Guy, 1976) scores, with subjects in the active treatment groups improving more than the placebo group. Several subsequent case studies, chart reviews, and open trials have demonstrated efficacy of neuroleptic treatment in both adults and adolescents as well. Spencer and colleagues (1995) reported on 19 children with schizophrenia between 5 and 11 years old who demonstrated consistent improvement using haloperidol (0.5 to 3.5 mg/day). Overall, studies of children and adolescents seem to indicate that about 70% of patients will show a good or partial response to antipsychotic drug treatment, although this may take 6–8 weeks to become apparent (Clark and Lewis, 1998).

The development of atypical antipsychotic agents has been a major advance in the pharmacotherapy of schizophrenia. In adult literature, atypical agents are at least as effective for positive symptoms and possibly more effective for negative symptoms as are typical neuroleptics (Meltzer et al., 1994). It is currently believed that this applies to child and adolescent schizophrenia as well (American Academy of Child and Adolescent Psychiatry, 2001). Additionally, the more favorable side effect profile of atypical agents often makes their use preferable to typical agents in the treatment of schizophrenia in children and adolescents (Toren, Ratner, Laor and Weizman, 2004). The use of risperidone in children and adolescents was examined in a case study of four schizophrenic patients between the ages of 12 and 18. These patients received risperidone (4 to 5 mg/day) for six months, and three of the four patients showed substantial improvement in negative symptoms with no side effects (Quintana and Keshavan, 1995). Risperidone use in adolescents was also studied in an open pilot study of ten adolescents between 11 and 18 years old. This study found clinically and statistically significant improvement on the Positive and Negative Syndrome Scale, the BPRS, and (CGI) at doses of 4.0 to 10.0 mg/day (Armenteros, Whitaker, Welikson, et al. 1997). Gothelf and colleagues (1995) evaluated the drug response of 43 adolescent patients treated with olanzapine, risperidone, or haloperidol for eight weeks in an open trial. They found that significant clinical improvement was seen by week four for all three treatment groups.

There are very limited data on treatment options beyond these aforementioned typical and atypical neuroleptics. However, some researchers suggest the use of adjuvant therapy (such as the addition of lithium, benzodiazepines, and anticonvulsants) or the use of ECT upon failure of such neuroleptic trials. Use of adjuvant therapies in youth with schizophrenia has not been studied, and even the evidence supporting its antipsychotic activity in adults is limited. Use of ECT in children has been described in several case reports with mixed results (Black, Wilcos, and Stewart, 1985; Kong and Glatter-Gotz, 1990; Willoughby, Hradek, and Richards, 1997). The AACAP practice parameters mention the use of ECT in treatment refractory cases, stating that the clinician must balance the relative risks and benefits of ECT against the morbidity of the disorder, the attitude of the patient and family, and the availability of other treatment options (American Academy of Child and Adolescent Psychiatry, 2001).

Defining treatment refractoriness

Defining treatment-refractoriness in schizophrenia is a difficult and controversial task. Because most patients experience persistent morbidity throughout their illness and full remissions are infrequent, the line between those who respond to treatment and those who do not can become blurred. Furthermore, although treatment resistance may occur from the onset of the illness, it more commonly develops over the course of the illness.

The most accepted criteria for defining treatment resistance in schizophrenia originates from the 1988 Multicenter Clozapine Trial (Kane, Honigsfeld, Singer et al. 1988). The following four criteria were used in this study to define refractoriness: persistent positive psychotic symptoms; current presence of at least moderately severe illness; persistence of illness with no stable period of good social and/or occupational functioning within the last five years; and at least three periods of treatment in the preceding five years with conventional antipsychotics at doses greater than 1000 mg per day chlorpromazine for 6 weeks, each without significant symptom relief and failure to improve by at least 20 percent in total BPRS score (Conley and Kelly, 2001). The treatment component of the criteria used by the Multicenter Clozapine Trial has been modified within the last few years in response to updated research. Treatment guidelines for defining treatment-resistance now state that, in addition to persistent positive features, current moderately severe illness, and persistent lack of social or occupational function, a patient must fail only two 4- to 6-week trials of 400–600 mg per day chlorpromazine in order to fulfill criteria for refractoriness (Barnes and McEvedy, 1996; Conley and Kelly, 2001).

Explanations for refractoriness

Prior to concluding that a child or adolescent with schizophrenia is treatment-refractory, several possibilities must first be considered. Poor treatment compliance, misdiagnosis of illness, inadequate duration of treatment, and inadequate dose of treatment are among issues that should be examined.

It should be noted that, although older adolescents were included in some of the studies described in the preceding section, the focus of these studies was on adults. Nonetheless, findings from other studies that focus on potentially correctible causes of treatment-refractoriness are applicable to young patients. Estimates of nonadherence to medication in schizophrenic patients range from 14 to 88 percent (Conley and Kelly, 2001). Patients who are nonadherent with medication have approximately a fourfold greater risk of relapse than those who are adherent. Therefore, in patients who are nonresponsive to medication and nonadherence is suspected, it may be worthwhile to attain a plasma level (Conley and Kelly, 2001). In cases where poor compliance is confirmed, prescription of a long-acting depot preparation is recommended. However, research on their usage specifically with young people has not yet been conducted (Clark and Lewis, 1998).

Treatment-refractoriness may be also be caused by misdiagnosis. This possibility has been explored primarily in adult studies, though it has been looked at in a few studies involving children and adolescents as well. Honer, Smith, MacEwan et al. (1994) assessed and rediagnosed (using DSM-III-R criteria) 110 severely and chronically ill adult patients with a referral diagnosis of schizophrenia. They found that the diagnosis of schizophrenia was confirmed in 80 patients (73 percent) but revised to another type of psychotic illness in 30 patients (27 percent). Patients with a revised diagnosis were less likely to receive neuroleptics and more likely to receive anti-mania drugs or ECT throughout their hospital stay. They were also less likely to require continued hospitalization on chronic care wards than those with confirmed schizophrenia. Smith, MacEwan, Ancill et al. (1992) conducted a similar study in which 50 consecutively admitted treatment-refractory psychotic adult patients were carefully reassessed using DSM-III-R criteria. Referral diagnoses were changed in 23 of the 50 patients. Patients whose diagnoses were changed were more likely to then receive mood-stabilizing medication and to show more improvement than those patients whose diagnosis did not change.

A limited number of studies investigating misdiagnosis as an explanation for treatment-refractoriness in children and adolescents have shown similar results as those with adults. One such study systematically examined a sample of 33 patients who were referred to a NIMH study of childhood-onset schizophrenia but who received research diagnoses of mood disorders instead by NIMH evaluation. Pilot data regarding the clinical course of these patients over a 2- to 7-year follow-up period showed that none of the subjects developed a clinical course resembling schizophrenia (Calderoni, Wudarsky, Bhangoo et al., 2001). Literature points to the fact that childhood syndromes, including bipolar disorder and psychotic depression, can be difficult to differentiate from schizophrenia (Hollis, 2000). Werry, McClellan, and Chard (1991) found that 25 percent of first-episode diagnoses of adolescent-onset schizophrenia were changed to bipolar disorder after five years. Clinicians and clinical researchers must take caution to effectively rule out psychotic mood disorders when making a diagnosis of schizophrenia, as children with mood disorders have been shown to respond well to mood-stabilizing and/or antidepressant medication (Calderoni et al., 2001).

Clozapine as treatment for otherwise refractory schizophrenia

Once a patient is duly determined to be refractory to other agents and all alternative explanations for this refractoriness have been explored, the most accepted next step is to initiate a trial of clozapine. Clozapine has virtually revolutionized the management of adults with treatment-refractory schizophrenia. Many published studies demonstrate its superiority over both typical and atypical agents in such cases (Avnon and Rabinowitz, 1995; Conley and Kelly, 2001; Chakos, Lieberman, Hoffman, et al. 2001; Azorin Spiegal, Remington et al., 2001; Ciapparelli Dell' Osso, Bandettini di Poggia et al., 2003). Studies have estimated that up to 60 percent of patients with otherwise refractory schizophrenia will respond to clozapine (Sharif, Raza & Ratakonda, 2000). Some studies have suggested that clozapine is even more effective when augmented with another atypical agent (Josiassen Joseph, Kohegyi et al., 2005). The APA reported, "the efficacy of clozapine over haloperidol in otherwise treatment-resistant cases has been clearly established in adults" (Clark and Lewis, 1998). Although its role is far less studied in the management of children and adolescents with treatment-refractory schizophrenia, available data largely indicate its efficacy in these subjects as well (Chalasani, Kant, and Chengappa, 2001). Of the atypical neuroleptics used in adolescents with schizophrenia, clozapine has been the most studied.

The overwhelming majority of published data describe the superiority of clozapine in treating schizophrenia with onset in childhood or adolescence. Kumra et al. (1996) compared clozapine to haloperidol in a six-week, double-blind, randomized study of children and adolescents with treatment-refractory schizophrenia. Clozapine-treated patients showed significantly more improvement in both positive and negative symptoms. Blanz and Schmidt (1993) looked at 57 schizophrenic adolescents treated with clozapine and found significant improvement in 67 percent and partial improvement in 21 percent. In another study, researchers used retrospective chart review to look at the effect of a clozapine trial on 21 inpatient nonresponders (12 of whom were under age 18). They found that there was a "marked improvement" in 11 patients and "some improvement" in six others (Armenteros et al., 1997). Another report found 10 out of 13 adolescent nonresponders to typical neuroleptics improved significantly with clozapine (Levkovitch, Kaysar, Kronnenberg, et al. 1994). Remschmidt, Fleischhaker and Hennighausen (2000) reviewed 15 studies that demonstrated the antipsychotic efficacy of clozapine in child and adolescent schizophrenia. They found that advantages of clozapine treatment in comparison with typical antipsychotics included higher antipsychotic efficacy during an acute schizophrenic episode, better improvement in chronic cases with a high load of negative symptoms, and fewer extrapyramidal side effects. Frazier et al. (1994) found that more than half of the 11 adolescents with childhood-onset schizophrenia showed marked improvement on BPRS ratings after a six-week open trial of clozapine.

Data also indicate that longer duration of treatment with clozapine tends to be more effective with treatment-refractory patients. In a 1999 meta-analysis of all available trial-based evidence on the effectiveness of clozapine in schizophrenia as compared with conventional neuroleptics, Wahlbeck, Cheine, Essali et al. (1999) found that, of the 30 included trials, seven included patients with treatment-refractory schizophrenia. These trials demonstrated that short-term (4–8 weeks) clozapine use in refractory patients was superior to conventional neuroleptics in terms of clinical improvement, BPRS scores, and negative symptom rating scales, but did not reveal any difference in relapse rates. Longer-term trials (10 weeks or longer) indicated superiority of clozapine in terms of clinical improvement, PANSS ratings, and relapse rates (Rosenheck et al., 1997; Buchanan, Breier, Kirkpatrick et al. 1998; Wahlbeck et al., 1999). Similarly, a 2003 double-blind, longitudinal study of treatment-resistant adults showed that although clozapine treatment of 12 weeks duration conferred statistically significant improvement in positive and negative symptoms when compared to typical antipsychotic medication, clozapine treatment of 6 weeks duration was not significantly different in effectiveness than typical antipsychotic medication. Researchers concluded that there is a need for prolonged treatment with clozapine to elicit its full effects on some treatment complexes (Lieberman, Safferman, Pollack et al., 1994; Pickar and Bartko, 2003).

Clozapine doesn't always work

Despite the strides that have been taken in the advent of clozapine as a treatment for resistant schizophrenia, it has only been found to be effective in about 30–50 percent of otherwise treatment-resistant patients (Kane, Honigfeld, Singer et al., 1988; Turetz, Mozes, Toren et al., 1997; Josiassen, Joseph, Kohegyi et al., 2005). Some studies suggest that clozapine is effective in up to 60 percent of refractory patients (Sharif, 1998). However, even generous estimates of clozapine's efficacy imply that there are many patients whose refractoriness extends even to clozapine.

As there are very limited data on almost all aspects of schizophrenia with onset in childhood or adolescence, it is not a surprise that the prevalence of treatment-refractoriness in this population has not been adequately assessed. Similarly, response rates to clozapine in such cases have not been well studied, and thus a great deal of uncertainty in the quantification of treatment-refractory schizophrenia occurring in adolescents remains. Without further research in this area, the management of treatment-refractory schizophrenia in this population is uncertain. Because schizophrenia with onset in childhood or adolescence tends to be more severe, more chronic, and more resistant to treatment than later-onset schizophrenia, it becomes particularly important to address the issue of treatment-refractoriness in the child and adolescent population. Although it is fairly accepted among clinicians that many children and adolescents with schizophrenia do present as refractory to medication, reports of such cases are virtually absent in current literature. This paper describes two patients seen in our center, with treatment given using the inpatient logic and experience of our center (most of which parallels many similar centers), and is not intended to be a new algorithm for treatment. We have described these two cases in an attempt both to illustrate the difficulty of the management of, and the profound need for further data regarding, adolescent treatment-refractory schizophrenia. Hopefully, with the emergence of such literature, better algorithms for treatment of these patients will emerge.

References

American Academy of Child and Adolescent Psychiatry (2001), Practice parameter for the assessment and treatment of children and adolescents with schizophrenia. *J. Amer. Acad. Child & Adolesc. Psychiat.*, 40:4S–23S.

Armenteros, J. L., Whitaker, A., H., Welikson, M., Stedge, D. J., & Gorman, J. (1997), Risperidone in adolescents with schizophrenia: An open pilot study. *J. Amer. Acad. Child & Adolesc. Psychiat.*, 36:694–700.

Avnon, M. & Rabinowitz, J. (1995), Effectiveness of clozapine in hospitalized people with chronic neuroleptic-resistant schizophrenia. *Brit. J. Psychiat.*, 167:760–764.

Azorin, J. M., Spiegel, R., Remington, G., Vanelle, J. M., Pere, J. J., Giguere, M., & Bourdeix, I. (2001), A double-blind comparative study of clozapine and risperidone in the management of severe chronic schizophrenia. *Amer. J. Psychiat.*, 158:1305–1313.

Barnes, T. R. & McEvedy, C. J. (1996), Pharmacological treatment strategies in the nonresponsive schizophrenic patient. *Int. Clin. Psychopharmacol.* 11(Suppl 2):67–71.

Beratis, S., Gabriel, J., & Hoidas, S. (1994), Age at onset in subtypes of schizophrenic disorders. *Schizophrenia Bull.* 20:287–296.

Black, D. W., Wilcox, J. A., & Stewart, M. (1985), The use of ECT in children: Case report. *J. Clin Psychiat.*, 46:98–99.

Blanz, B. & Schmidt, M. (1993), Clozapine for schizophrenia (letter). *J. Amer. Acad. Child & Adolesc. Psychiat.*, 32:223–224.

Buchanan, R. W., Breier, A., Kirkpatrick, B., Ball, P., & Carpenter, W. T., Jr. (1998), Positive and negative symptom response to clozapine in schizophrenic patients with and without the deficit syndrome. *Amer. J. Psychiat.*, 155:751–760.

Calderoni, D., Wudarsky, M., Bhangoo, R., Dell, M. L., Nicolson, R., Hamburger, S. D., Gochman, P., Lenane, M., Rapoport, J. L., & Leibenluft, C. (2001), Differentiating childhood-onset schizophrenia from psychotic mood disorders. *J. Amer. Acad. Child & Adolesc. Psychiat.*, 40:1190–1196.

Chakos, M., Lieberman, J., Hoffman, E., Bradford, D., & Sheitman, B. (2001), Effectiveness of second-generation antipsychotics in patients with treatment-resistant schizophrenia: A review and meta-analysis of randomized trials. *Amer. J. Psychiat.*, 158:518–526.

Chalasani, L., Kant, R., & Chengappa, K. N. (2001), Clozapine impact on clinical outcomes and aggression in severely ill adolescents with childhood-onset schizophrenia. *Can. J. Psychiat.*, 46:965–968.

Ciapparelli, A., Dell'Osso, L., Bandettini di Poggia, A., Carmassi, C., Cecconi, D., Fenzi, M., Chiavacci M. C., Bottai, M., Ramacciotti, C. E., & Cassano, G. B. (2003), Clozapine in treatment-resistant patients with schizophrenia, schizoaffective disorder, or psychotic bipolar disorder: A naturalistic 48-month follow-up study. *J. Clin Psychiat.*, 64(4):451–458.

Clark, A. F. & Lewis, S. W. (1998), Practitioner review: Treatment of schizophrenia in childhood and adolescence. *J. Child Psychol. Psychiat.*, 39:1071–1081.

Conley, R. R. & Kelly, D. L. (2001), Management of treatment resistance in schizophrenia. *Biol Psychiat.*, 50:898–911.

Frazier, J. A., Gordon, C. T., McKenna, K., Lenane, M. C., Jih, D., & Rapoport, J. L. (1994), An open trial of clozapine in 11 adolescents with childhood-onset schizophrenia. *J. Amer. Acad. Child & Adolesc. Psychiat.*, 33:658–663.

Guy, W. (1976). Clinical global impressions. In *ECDEU Assessment Manual for Psychopharmacology*, revised (DHEW Publ No ADM 76–338). Rockville, MD: National Institute of Mental Health, pp. 218–222.

Hafner, H., & Nowotny, B. (1995), Epidemiology of early-onset schizophrenia. *Eur. Arch. Psychiat. Clin. Neurosci.*, 245:80–90.

Hollis, C. (2000), Adult outcomes of child- and adolescent-onset schizophrenia: Diagnostic stability and predictive validity. *Amer. J. Psychiat.*, 157:1652–1659.

Honer, W. G., Smith, G. N., MacEwan, G. W., Kopala, L., Altman, S., Yorkston, N., Ehmann, T. S., Smith, A., & Lang, M. (1994), Diagnostic reassessment and treatment response in schizophrenia. *J. Clin. Psychiat.*, 55: 528–532.

Jacobsen, L. K. & Rapoport, J. L. (1998), Childhood-onset schizophrenia: Implications of clinical and neurobiological research. *J. Child Psychol Psychiat.,* 39:101–113.

Josiassen, R. C., Joseph, A., Kohegyi, E., Stokes, S., Dadvand, M., Paing, W. W., & Shaughnessy, R. A. (2005), Clozapine augmented with risperidone in the treatment of schizophrenia: A randomized, double-blind, placebo-controlled trial. *Amer. J. Psychiat.,* 162:130–136.

Kane, J., Honigfeld, G., Singer, J., & Meltzer, H. (1988), Clozapine for the treatment-resistant schizophrenic: A double-blind comparison with chlorpromazine. *Arch Gen Psychiat.,* 45:789–796.

Kong, P. & Glatter-Gotz, U. (1990), Combined electroconvulsive and neuroleptic therapy in schizophrenia refractory to neuroleptics. *Schizophr. Res.,* 3:351–354.

Kravariti, E., Morris, R. G., Rabe-Hesketh, S., Murray, R. M., & Frangou, S. (2003), The Maudsley early onset schizophrenia study: Cognitive function in adolescents with recent onset schizophrenia. *Schizophrenia Research,* 61:137–148.

Kumra, S., Frazier, J. A, Jaconsen, L. K., McKenna, K., Gordon, C. T., Lenane, M. C., Hamburger, S. D., Smith, A. K., Albus, K. E., Alaghband-Rad, J., & Rapoport, J. L. (1996), Childhood-onset schizophrenia: A double-blind clozapine-haloperidol comparison. *Arch Gen Psychiat.,* 53: 1090–1097.

Kumra, S., Jacobsen, L. K., Lenane, M., Karp, B. I., Frazier, J. A, Smith, A. K., Bedwell, J., Lee, P., Malanga, C. J., Hamburger, S., & Rapoport, J. L. (1998), Childhood-onset schizophrenia: An open-label study of olanzapine in adolescents. *J. Amer. Acad. Child & Adolesc. Psychiat.,* 37:377–385.

Kumra, S., Shaw, M., Merka, P., Nakayama, E., & Augustin, R. (2001), Childhood-onset schizophrenia: Research update. *Can. J. Psychiat.,* 46:923–930.

Levkovitch, Y., Kaysar, N., Kronnenberg, Y., Hagai, H., & Gaoni, B. (1994), Clozapine for schizophrenia (letter). *J. Amer. Acad. Child & Adolesc. Psychiat.,* 33:431.

Lieberman, J. A., Safferman, A. Z., Pollack, S., Szymanski, S., Johns, C., Howard, A., Kronig, M., Bookstein, P., & Kane, J. M. (1994), Clinical effects of clozapine in chronic schizophrenia: Response to treatment and predictors of outcome. *Amer. J. Psychiat.,* 151:1744–1752.

Loranger, A. W. (1984), Sex differences in age of onset of schizophrenia. *Arch. Gen. Psychiat.,* 41:157–161.

Meltzer, H. Y. (1997), Treatment-resistant schizophrenia: The role of clozapine. *Curr. Med, Res, Opin.,* 14:1–20.

Meltzer, H. Y., Lee, M. A., & Ranjan, R. (1994), Recent advances in the pharmacotherapy of schizophrenia. *Acta Psychiatr. Scand.,* 90(suppl 384):95–101.

Overall, J. E. and Gorham, D. R. (1962). The brief psychiatric rating scale. *Psychol. Rep.,* 10:790–812.

Pickar, D. & Bartko J. J. (2003), Effect size of symptom status in withdrawal of typical antipsychotics and subsequent clozapine treatment in patients with treatment-resistant schizophrenia. *Amer. J. Psychiat.,* 160:1133–1138.

Pool, D., Bloom, W., Mielke, D.H., Roniger, J. J. Jr, Gallant, D. M. (1976) A controlled evaluation of loxitane in seventy-five adolescent schizophrenic patients. *Curr. Ther. Res. Clin. Exp.* 19:99–104.

Quintana, H. & Keshavan, M. (1995), Risperidone in children and adolescents with schizophrenia. *J. Amer. Acad. Child & Adolesc. Psychiat.,* 34:1292–1296.

Remschmidt, H., Fleischhaker, C., Hennighausen, K., & Schultz, E. (2000), Management of schizophrenia in children and adolescents. *Paediatric Drugs,* 2: 253–262.

Remschmidt, H. E., Schultz, E., Martin, M., Warnke, A., & Trott, G. E. (1994), Childhood-onset schizophrenia: History of the concept and recent studies. *Schizophrenia Bull.,* 20:727–745.

Rosenheck, R., Cramer, J., Xu, W., Thomas, J., Henderson, W., Frisman, L., Fye, C., & Charney, D. (1997), A comparison of clozapine and haloperidol in hospitalized patients with refractory schizophrenia. *N. Engl. J. Med.,* 337:809–815.

Sharif, Z. A. (1998), Treatment refractory schizophrenia: How should we proceed? *Psychiatr. Q.,* 69:263–281.

Sharif, Z. A., Raza, A., & Ratakonda, S. S. (2000), Comparative efficacy of risperidone and clozapine in the treatment of patients with refractory schizophrenia or schizoaffective disorder: A retrospective analysis. *J. Clin Psychiat.,* 61:498–504.

Sheitman, B. B. & Lieberman, J. A. (1998), The natural history and pathophysiology of treatment resistant schizophrenia. *J. Psychiatric Res.,* 32:143–150.

Smith, G. N., MacEwan, G. W., Ancill, R. J., Honer, W. G., & Ehmann, T. S. (1992), Diagnostic confusion in treatment-refractory psychotic patients. *J. Clin Psychiat.,* 53:197–200.

Toren, P., Ratner, S., Laor, N., & Weizman, A. (2004), Benefit-risk assessment of atypical antipsychotics in the treatment of schizophrenia and comorbid disorders in children and adolescents. *Drug Safety,* 27:1135–56.

Turetz, M., Mozes, T., Toren, P., Chernauzan, N., Yoran-Hegesh, R., Mester, R., Wittenberg, N., Tyano, S., & Weizman, A. (1997), An open trial of clozapine in neuroleptic-resistant childhood-onset schizophrenia. *Brit J. Psychiat.,* 170:507–510.

Wahlbeck, K., Cheine, M., Essali, A., & Adams, C. (1999), Evidence of clozapine's effectiveness in schizophrenia: A systematic review and meta-analysis of randomized trials. *Amer. J. Psychiat.,* 156:990–999.

Werry, J. S., McClellan, J. M., & Chard, L. (1991), Childhood and adolescent schizophrenia, bipolar and schizoaffective disorders: A clinical and outcome study. *J. Amer. Acad. Child & Adolesc. Psychiat.,* 30:457–465.

Willoughby, C. L., Hradek, E. A., & Richards, N. R. (1997), Use of electroconvulsive therapy with children: An overview and case report. *J. Child Adolesc. Psychiatr. Nurs.,* 10:11–17.

Yang, P. C., Liu, C. Y., Chiang, S. Q., Chen, J. Y., & Lin, T. S. (1995), Comparison of adult manifestations of schizophrenia with onset before and after 15 years of age. *Acta Psychiatr. Scand.,* 91:209–212.

15 We Do Not Need to Throw Out the Baby with the Bath Water

Discussion of "When Clozapine doesn't work"

Max Sugar

Discussion

The paper by Stahl, Shapiro, Hertzig, and Turchin (2007, chapter 14, this volume) represents one side of the dilemma of many psychiatrists at present. With the increased focus on the biological aspects of behavior and the availability of a wider array of psychopharmacological agents, there are marked differences in approaches to, and expectations from, psychiatric therapy for many conditions. In their paper, the focus is on the pharmacological.

The authors are to be commended for the great effort involved in their therapeutic endeavors. Although the authors indicate that 20 to 33 percent of all schizophrenics are resistant to pharmacotherapy, and that 30 to 60 percent of patients do not respond to clozapine, they seem to feel disappointed and surprised that clozapine, the drug of last resort, did not cure or improve their schizophrenic adolescents. Yet, should we not recall that in the field of medicine we rarely cure, we sometimes help, but we can always comfort?

The anamnesis has a striking paucity of information about the youngsters' development, early history, family history, conflicts, and behavioral problems until the onset of their illness. A noncontributory history in a psychotic patient raises many questions and notions about such things as denial, avoidance, family secrets, trauma, scapegoating, the double-bind, and so on. Assessment of neglect and abuse (both physical and sexual) of children and adolescents needs to be considered as part of a psychiatric evaluation.

It would have been helpful to better understand the cases if there were more clarity about some other particulars. There is no agreement in the literature about early-onset schizophrenia since it has been defined variously, as the authors note. Had they focused on the onset of schizophrenia in adolescence, it would have avoided the blurring of definitions and confusion about the topic. We need to recall that schizophrenia was originally termed "dementia praecox," due to its frequent onset in adolescence. Although two adolescents are the basis for the paper, the authors do not limit their inquiry and literature review to that developmental period. By including child and adult schizophrenics, and combining children with adolescents in a review of treatment, a confounding occurs.

An algorithm for treatment of refractory schizophrenia would have been useful to understand the authors' approaches to these patients. Such an algorithm would help to explain the dosages used and choices of the various medications; the decision to perform ECT; the rationale for using stimulants with serotonin reuptake inhibitors (SSRIs); and the strategy of augmenting with olanzapine instead of switching to an alternative monotherapy. Did the authors consider using some of the pretranquilizer therapies, which were often very helpful in treating schizophrenia, such as hydrotherapy, along with pharmacotherapy and psychotherapy?

Interestingly, there is no mention of a psychotherapeutic effort by the authors, as if it is passé. Did they make efforts to initiate individual or group psychotherapy, or family therapy, or establish a therapeutic alliance? Understandably, that takes time and a lot of effort with a patient with schizophrenia. Perhaps issues of insurance limits and the hope of a rapid response to medication kept such notions off their therapeutic radar. A few very brief case reports might help make the point that psychotherapy should not be overlooked.

Case example #1

In the course of treating a psychotic 10-year-old male, I met the mother only once—in the initial interviews with the father. Thereafter, the father brought the boy to the therapy sessions. When I casually wondered about the mother's situation some time later, the father's reply was noncommittal. After many months of therapy, when the youngster began making considerable progress, the father informed me that the mother had been in the state hospital for a while with a psychosis. The lad continued to improve, and eventually was discharged from treatment. It seemed that part of his successful outcome was due to his no longer being the symptom-carrier for the mother's psychosis. Or perhaps, as therapy helped him, he no longer passively accepted mother's infliction of trauma, which altered the family dynamics and exposed her illness.

Case example #2

After an 18-year-old female U.S. Marine private was diagnosed as a paranoid schizophrenic, her diary and letters to her commanding officer, a major, were found to contain many references about the major. These were rambling writings about being forced into homosexual activities with her and other superior officers, and served to confirm her delusional condition. Soon after she enlisted, the major had recruited this very talented athlete to be on her women marines' baseball team, which she coached. The coach had been lauded for the team's marked success in winning the championship of all the military services a few months earlier, so that she appeared above reproach. Several months later the major and all the officers and noncommissioned officers on the baseball team were court-martialed for homosexuality and forcing those under their command into homosexual activities with them.

Case example #3

This 16-year-old male inpatient, who was diagnosed as a borderline personality disorder, distrusted everyone. This made his therapy progress very slowly, but after a long period in therapy he developed a therapeutic alliance. He then divulged that his older brother had forced him into homosexual activities for several years until admission to the hospital. His brother had made him promise to never reveal this, and threatened him with retaliation if he did. When he informed his parents of this in family therapy, they reacted with hostile surprise, disbelief, followed by guilt. Thereafter, his therapy progressed more suitably and successfully.

Case example #4

This youngster's alcoholic and neglectful parents died when she was in the Oedipal stage. Then she was raised by relatives who enjoyed the considerable largesse of her inheritance, but continued to neglect her. Accordingly, her ego development was obstructed. Left to her own devices, she wandered into adolescence with little guidance and then into the "hippie" scene of the '70s, which led to many "trips" and acting out. After her misconduct eventuated in jail or rehab, she saw many psychiatrists for varying periods as an outpatient and inpatient with the diagnosis of schizophrenia. In her last hospitalization she was routinely unkempt and disheveled. Due to tranquilizers she was lethargic but her acting out was controlled. She seemed headed for the back ward of a state hospital, but for a large trust fund, which provided extremely well for her private care.

After the retirement of her admitting psychiatrist she was referred to another psychiatrist with an interest in psychotherapy. Following a change in psychotropics, her lethargy ended. Then a therapeutic relationship evolved very slowly. Eventually, she was able to leave the hospital, live in her own apartment with a caretaker, continue with her treatment, and even go shopping, and out to dinner with her nurse-companion.

A review of some past psychotherapeutic endeavors with schizophrenic patients in the writings of Paul Federn (1943), Frieda Fromm-Reichmann (1950), Lewis Hill (1973), Marguerite Sechehaye (1951a), and Gertrud Schwing (1954) would perhaps help to reassess psychotherapy with schizophrenics as significant, along with the judicious use of tranquilizers. The books *I Never Promised You a Rose Garden* (Greenberg, 1964) and *Autobiography of a Schizophrenic Girl* (Sechehaye, 1951b) provide a view of the illness and psychoanalytic treatment from the patient's standpoint.

The works of Beckett et al. (1956) and Johnson, Giffin, Watson, and Beckett (1956) merit a reappraisal in terms of the genesis of schizophrenia. Although Adelaide Johnson and her coworkers (1956) agreed that delusions of the schizophrenic contain powerful instinctual components, "the initial schizophrenic delusion is largely an expression, albeit disguised, of the overwhelming exogenous trauma which the patient has experienced ... with striking specificity represents a life experience of the patient" (pp. XX). The parents of Johnson's patients had treatment with members of her research team, and the team members worked collaboratively. From these efforts they found a history of exogenous trauma consisting of 1) persistent obstruction to ego development and 2) discrete physical or psychological assault.

The work of Ross Speck and Carolyn Attneave (1973) presents some similar ideas on a larger scale. The "network therapy" that Speck initiated helps realign the dynamics in the patient's relationship network by exposing the puppeteer who exercises a malignant influence on the behavior and feelings of the patient and others in the network. The puppeteer uses others to scapegoat, avoid, deny, evade, and keep secrets in order to control them and the patient. The patient becomes the symptom-bearer for the network's pathology. With the exposure of the puppeteer in network therapy, changes occur in the network alignments, and the designated patient no longer is the puppet who endorses the pathology of the puppeteer and the network.

Sugar (1971) introduced the use of "self-selected adolescent peer group therapy" for adolescents facing imminent hospitalization due to a severe crisis, suicidal feelings, or other reasons. The information that the peers provided about the patient's problems and his/her behavior contributed to a resolution of the crisis, which avoided hospitalization.

Sugar, Stuckey, and Garrett (1971) and Sugar (1975) described a successful therapeutic research project that helped avoid hospitalization of psychotic latency-age children. This was done with a college-student ombudsman who was in each child's home for a significant number of hours each week. During this time the ombudsman observed repeated trauma inflicted on the child by the parent(s). The presence of the ombudsman disrupted this. His/her sharing this information in supervision, and the resultant use of the data in the family or individual sessions with the parents led to a change in family dynamics and parental behavior. This relieved the child from being the symptom-carrier for the family, and avoided hospitalization of the child.

This brief outline of some psychotherapeutic approaches to schizophrenia does not exhaust the list of contributors. We should not overlook the fact that schizophrenia is best considered as a group of psychoses, i.e., with subtypes. Psychogenomics may elucidate the differences in the group of schizophrenias, and clarify which type responds best to which therapy.

Perhaps this paper by Stahl and collegues in this volume may become a stimulus for the reconsideration of a broader framework for psychiatric treatment of adolescent schizophrenia. This would include individual, family, and collaborative psychotherapy, group therapy, network therapy, self-selected adolescent peer group psychotherapy, and psychopharmacology.

About the Author

Dr. Sugar was president of the American Society for Adolescent Psychiatry in 1973–74. He was Editor-in Chief of The Annals of Adolescent Psychiatry, 1982–85. Dr. Sugar is Emeritus Professor of Clinical Psychiatry at Louisiana State University Medical Center, Department of Psychiatry in New Orleans, LA.

References

Beckett, P. G. S., Robinson, D. B., Frazier, S. H., Steinhilber, R. M., Duncan, G. M., Estes, H. R., Litin, E. M., Grattan, R. T., & Johnson, A. M. (1956), The significance of exogenous traumata in the genesis of schizophrenia. *Psychiatry*, 19:137–142.

Federn, P. (1943), Psychoanalysis of psychoses. *Psychiatric Quart.*, 17:3–19.

Fromm-Reichmann, F. (1950), *Principles of Intensive Psychotherapy.* Chicago: University of Chicago Press.

Greenberg, J. (1964), *I Never Promised You a Rose Garden.* New York: Penguin Books.

Hill, L. B. (1973), *Psychotherapeutic Intervention in Schizophrenia.* Chicago: University of Chicago Press.

Johnson, A. M., Giffin, M. E., Watson, J., & Beckett, P. G. S. (1956), Observations on ego functions in schizophrenia. *Psychiatry*, 19:143–148.

Schwing, G. (1954), *A Way to the Soul of the Mentally Ill.* New York: International Universities Press.

Sechehaye, M. A. (1951a), *Symbolic Realization: A New Method of Psychotherapy Applied to a Case of Schizophrenia,* trans. B. Wursten & H. Wursten. New York: International Universities Press.

Sechehaye, M. (1951b), *Autobiography of a Schizophrenic Girl; With Analytic Interpretation by Marguerite Sechehaye,* trans. G. Rubin-Rabson. New York: Grune & Stratton.

Speck, R. & Attneave, C. (1973), *Family Networks.* New York: Pantheon Books.

Stahl, A. S., Shapiro, T., Hertzig, M. E., & Turchin, W. (2007), When clozapine doesn't work: Two case reports of treatment-refractory adolescent schizophrenia. In: *Adolescent Psychiatry*, vol. 30, ed. L. T. Flaherty. Mahwah, NJ: Analytic Press, pp. 179–192.

Sugar, M. (1971), Network psychotherapy of an adolescent. *Adolescent Psychiatry,* 1:464–478.

_____ (1975), Use of college-student companions for psychotic children to avoid hospitalization. *J. Amer. Acad. Child & Adolesc. Psychiat.*, 14:249–267.

_____, Stuckey, B. & Garrett, M. (1971), Group supervision of student companions to psychotic children. *Internat. J. Group Psychother.*, 21:301–309.

16 Drs. Stahl et al. respond to Dr. Sugar's discussion

Atara S. Stahl, Theodore Shapiro, Margaret E. Hertzig, Wendy Turchin

Response

Although negative responses to treatment are rampant, they are infrequently recorded in the literature. Insofar as many of our seriously ill adolescents are at risk for chronic courses, especially in the schizophrenic group, we decided to report on the two cases that were well documented in our files. The report happens to come at a time when we have pharmacologic agents that do alter the course for some patients and we also know that psychosocial interventions (including various psychotherapies) may be adjunctive but alone are relatively useless, Mme. Sechehaye and Frieda Fromm-Reichman notwithstanding. Although many of us grew up in psychiatry reading such cases and were impressed and enlightened about how the mind of the schizophrenic works, these cases remain dubious in their continuing relevance to our contemporary search for relief and improved adaptation. Currently, the focus on pharmacological agents alone or in company of other psychological supports seems to be the most promising avenue.

We are remiss, however, in not describing the variety of psychological supports that are part of our usual in-patient milieu and the associated group and family work that were employed in the cases that we described. Indeed, our orientation at the Payne Whitney Clinic is multimodal, and there is a distinctively psycho-dynamic approach to our case formulations. True, none of this is spelled out in our case histories. Nor is the singular psychotherapeutic work that was done in the first case.

In response to Dr. Sugar's inquiry regarding mixing early-onset with late-onset schizophrenia in our report of the literature, we do so because these cases both had suspected onsets prior to clinical encounter. This is as reflected in pre- and early adolescent disruption leading to some medical intervention in the first case and removal from the home to an uncle in the suburbs and a less pressured academic environment in the second. It was also the case that intellectual and academic deterioration, as seen with classical dementia praecox, did not occur until late adolescence in these cases. We thought that was relevant to the course and to our fellow psychiatrists looking toward prognosis in their schizophrenic adolescents.

In a time when hospitals are designed for treatment and patients are no longer "warehoused" in state hospitals, it is important for clinicians to realize that we do not help all our patients, save curing any. The final reason for this report is that the pendulum of diagnosing schizophrenia may have swung too far to the pole of missing the diagnosis due to the reluctance of young clinicians to make the diagnosis. Bipolarity seems to be preferred because there is a plausible treatment with more hope. Though we should not err on the side of despair, we must also be must be alert to the significance of better diagnoses as a guide to treatment. There are recent data to support that if schizophrenia is diagnosed in its prodromal phases, some frank breakdowns may be aborted (McGorry et al, 2002).

This clinical report is merely a cautionary tale concerning a reality that is somewhat difficult to accept, which is that some cases are less responsive to all our efforts and continue to require our scrutiny. Just as chlorpromazine and the older neuroleptics have been replaced by the newer generation neuroleptics including clozapine, we may expect that new pharmacologic agents may soon be on the horizon. This does not preclude the reintroduction of other psychotherapeutic efforts that make adolescents more tractable, amenable to education, and adaptive despite their schizophrenias.

References

McGorry, P. D., Yung, A. R., Phillips, L. J., Yuen, H. P., Francey, S., Cosgrave, E. M., Germano, D., Bravin, J., McDonald, T., Blair, A., Adlard, S., & Jackson, H. (2002), Randomized controlled trial of interventions designed to reduce the risk of progression to first-episode psychosis in a clinical sample with subthreshold symptoms. *Arch. Gen. Psychiatr.*, 59:921–926.

Index

C

T - #0526 - 101024 - C0 - 229/152/13 - PB - 9781138005921 - Gloss Lamination